"Terrific book; easy to read a
—*Dr. John Walker, Professo.*
American College of Sports Medicine

"This book will change your life. If you are starting on your weight loss journey, this book teaches you little things such as eating every two hours, how to plan your meal, importance of exercise...It is the most honest and genuine book where the intention clearly is to help people and change the way they think about WEIGHT LOSS."
—*Professor Inderjit Kaur, YWCA, India*

"If the heart is willing, this is the choice for victory!"
—*Pastor Rusty Martin, Island Church, Galveston, TX*

"Dr Willis has provided an informative and easy-to-follow book. It provides the relevant detail to those readers who want to change their behavior to food and exercise in the search for achieving weight loss. The book has three sections and presents 18 chapters in all. Section one provides a clear foundation—asking those questions many of us ask, whilst the second section prepares you to change for the better. Section three focuses on exercise in its early chapters but concentrates on top steps and useful recipes in later chapters. Throughout the book is supported with useful photos and diagrams and the ethos of RightSize from food forecasting (and portion size) to energy surge exercises. This is an excellent read and companion for those individuals wishing to following a sensible program that provides a guide to a sustained healthy weight loss."
—*Dr. Sarah Curran, Cardiff Metropolitan University (Wales, UK), Royal College of Physicians and Surgeons of Glasgow*

RightSize Weight Loss™

Metabolism acceleration for easy weight loss
without strenuous exercise or a rigid diet

Dr. FB Willis, CPL, BA, MEd, MBBS, PhD, FACSM

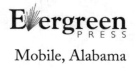

E ergreen
PRESS

Mobile, Alabama

Evergreen Press
P.O. Box 191540 • Mobile, AL 36619
800-367-8203

CONTENTS

Section I. New Lives from Weight Loss

Brief Overview   *1*

1. Experiences of RightSizing   *3*
2. Simple Adjustments   *12*
3. Why Other Programs Fail   *16*
4. Easy, Natural, Permanent Change   *21*
5. Where Are You Now?   *27*

Section II. Activate Your Energy Surge

6. Ignite Your Metabolism   *40*
7. Natural Foods for Higher Energy   *54*
8. Eat Often for Better Digestion   *64*
9. Let's Get Real   *69*
10. Tease, not Overload   *77*
11. Activate the Change   *82*

Section III. Your Best Body Forever

12. Muscle Stretching   *90*
13. Exercise Phys-E-O!   *106*
14. Proof for the Professional   *111*
15. Top Steps   *134*
16. Scripture   *138*
17. Support for Success   *143*

Bibliography   *150*
Body Summation Score   *159*

This book is dedicated to my Savior
who saved and saves me!
It is also dedicated to my loving parents,
Frank and Georgia Willis. My mom taught me
how to say "Can do!" even in the most challenging circumstances,
and my Dad showed me how to use a methodical
approach like using the compass and square
so that I am duly and truly prepared!
Thanks to my family and Jesus!

Introduction

I designed a revolutionary, easy and flexible protocol to help my friends feel like the beautiful people they are to me! My formula has been responsible for helping people reduce pounds and inches to acquire and maintain the RightSize body for each one! (Most people are not meant to be a "skinny mini.") Today, over 200 million Americans and 1.6 billion people in the world are categorically overweight, and the RightSize program will change the world's waistline with this amazingly easy, three option plan. I prescribe either a set portion-size serving with more frequent eating for the fastest digestion, a brief Energy Surge exercise before eating, or eating only natural foods (comes from the earth not a factory).

Good news! This book will give you the exact, effective formula that you can use in every situation, any circumstance, and at any time to lose weight and sizes quickly. It is our responsibility to care for our bodies as the holiest of temples (1 Cor. 3:16). Together let's say, "Eat cake and lose weight!" as we achieve our RightSize and glorify God!

After experiencing what the FAA described as an "unsurvivable (uncontrollable) plane crash," I endured a 36-month series of 16 sequential operations to rebuild my legs, so I know what it is like to be so weak that I couldn't even hold up my own weight up. The pain from a bone infection left me often praying to "go home to Jesus." During this time, though, God empowered me to start earning four more degrees (including a medical degree from a university in the British Commonwealth and PhD in kinesiology).

As a result, I dedicated my life to helping others overcome their physical challenges. After leading powerful, international research for ten years, I was given a lifetime achievement when I was chosen to be a Fellow of the American College of Sports Medicine (FACSM). My research has been presented research at dozens of national and international medical conferences with accreditation as a lecturer in continuing medical education.

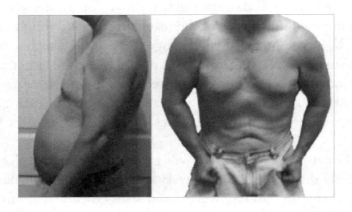

Empathy is one part of my mission because I found myself to be overweight after forty (224 lbs.). After refining the formula to RightSize myself, I have maintained a healthy 180 lbs. Professionally I have owned and operated successful health/rehab/fitness centers in the US and Caribbean to help achieve accelerated weight loss. Teaching undergraduates has also been a blessing because my heart is to be an uplifting, empowering clinician, coach, and cheerleader who says, "Never worry about your waistline again!"

SECTION I

New Lives from Weight Loss

A Brief Overview

Today our world is suffering the greatest epidemic of obesity in history, and our health care costs and death rates are both rising. Two thirds of our country are overweight, including 40% who are categorically obese. Do you remember when we used to pride ourselves that our country was the fittest in the world? People are trying to become more fit by spending over 20 billion dollars a year in the US for weight loss, but the current efforts are not working.

The RightSize program offers a simple, holistic, flexible program with three options that people can use to obtain their RightSize physique quickly and keep that stature for a lifetime. This is done by using one or more of three flexible tools (PEN) for each dining event. PEN stands for **P**ortion size (eating small portions five to six times per day), **E**nergy Surge (revving up one's heartbeat just before eating), or **N**atural Nutrition (eating non-processed foods).

In a nutshell, the first option of consuming a limited **Portion** size allows for faster digestion by giving us smaller amounts to eat more often. In the second option, brief, **Energy Surge** exercises elevate the heart rate for 2-3 minutes before eating, thereby increasing the metabolism so food is broken down for use as fuel and not deposited as fat. The third option of using **Natural Nutrition** means eating un-packaged, unprocessed whole foods that accelerates our di-gestion because our body does not have to deal with foreign chemicals. This quicker digestion prevents accumulation of fat.

The principle cause of so many Americans being over-weight is that we are eating too many foods that are filled with chemical preservatives that often have cancer causing additives. Plus we don't exercise as people used to do. How many children were overweight 100 years ago? They ran, played, worked on the farm, and ate natural foods that did not include cancer causing chemicals like TBHQ, a preserva-tive that is in most packaged foods.

This book describes how to use the easy PEN formula as soon as you wake up to start regaining your RightSize before you are even out of bed. When were you in your best shape? Let's make that answer "later this year!" You don't need a gym or equipment for this program. All it takes is a few minutes a day of brief, unique exercise, and "forecasting your food" to quickly acquire your RightSize! The RightSize program has been responsible for reducing thousands of inches for people who could not lose weight from other programs. This book will yield millions of new success stories from readers who will RightSize their bodies. Let's start your success story today!

1

Experiences of RightSizing

"I had tried ten diet plans from age 24 to 44 with roller coaster effects until I quit trying, and I became even heavier. It was not until I met Doc Willis who helped me design my unique formula that gave me quick success. Now I can binge at Christmas and still lose weight, as long as it was preceded with a quick three minutes of a unique exercise. Not only have I lost 55 pounds in five years but even more importantly, I now have helped my daughter avoid the roller coaster weights! Doc taught me to be a victor not a victim!" *(Raelyn A., Austin, Texas)*

RightSize Victors!

Jill was a tall, beautiful, statuesque woman in her early thirties. However, she retained substantial weight from her last pregnancy. She tried several other weight loss programs that were not unsuccessful. She set the goal to return to her college dress size in nine months, and she began this program while wearing dress size 20. After medical screening, she had her body composition measured with the BodPod testing chamber, and my assistant calculated her Body Summation score (more about that later). She started with the PEN program (Portion Size, Energy Surge, or Natural Nutrition), and she achieved a 20% decrease of body fat in just 30 days. This encouraged her to share this goal with her family.

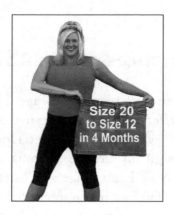

Size 20
to Size 12
in 4 Months

To begin implementing her new regimen, Jill came up with the plan that before lunch she would take her kids to the park, and they would all run across the fields together. Quick, playful runs with her kids gave her the Energy Surge before eating. She also became passionate about eating all organic foods which "keep the fire high" rather than eating cheap, "low flame" foods. She also loved using TIPS throughout the day. (TIPS equals Tease-eating Increases Powerful Stimulation for your metabolism, which raises your body's energy level through the roof—more about that later).

After nine months, her body fat percentage had been cut in half, and Jill went from size 20 to 12, which was her college dress size! She simply used the PEN formula to regain her RightSize for a lifetime of fitness and beauty! After ten years, now she is size 8/10!

Disability Overcome with Doc's Program

Karen was forced to seek temporary disability because of obesity and Chronic Obstructive Pulmonary Disease (COPD). She was unable to work in an office for eight hours and then drive home without being acutely fatigued. After a week's work, she would often be sick all weekend. Karen was 40 years old, 260 lbs., 5'2" tall, and her Body Mass Index (BMI) was over 40 (body weight in pounds ÷ height in inches x 10). This is considered to be "morbid obesity." She had been a smoker for 20 years, starting in college. Her chest often felt tight and left her short of breath (but she had no acute heart illness). After being infected with chronic bronchitis for two months, she sadly was forced to file for disability leave.

Before consulting me, she had tried pharmaceutical products, which were not effective for her weight loss, and she was also pre-diabetic. Her health condition looked grave. In the first phone call, I advised her to start moving while still in bed. In our second phone call, I gave Karen the plan that showed her a glimpse of her future fitness. I encouraged her and helped her say and believe in the words, "Can do!"

She began a motion with her back on the bed, her legs in midair, moving them as if she were pedaling a bicycle. She lay on her back with her feet above her torso and pedaled as if the bike were above her. She counted how many minutes she could do that before becoming fatigued. At first she could only air pedal for two minutes, but soon she was able to continue for ten minute intervals. She was excited when she began doing these three times a day but knew that she needed more of a challenge. Karen was embarrassed to go to the wellness center because she was still morbidly obese. She bought an indoor bicycle and then began increasing her minutes and frequency of riding.

After two months, Karen felt so much better that she asked to return to her workplace. Her colleagues remarked how much better she looked, and she proudly said that the PEN program gave her "endurance for life!" Over the next few years Karen increased her consumption of natural foods for five meals a day that propelled her weight loss of 88 pounds, before completing her first 100-mile bicycle ride! She joyfully brags that the PEN formula has helped her regain her RightSize!

Mommy Tummy NO MORE!

Amy, a friend of Karen's saw her success, which inspired her to work toward losing weight too. Amy said that she was never able to lose her pregnancy fat even though she exercised and watched what she ate. I had her complete the "Let's Get Real Survey" (see chapter 9) and saw that she was eating healthy food but at almost six hour intervals (6am – noon – and 7 pm). I also saw that Rachel's exercise was too intense because a lower intensity ride uses fat as fuel. I placed Amy on a 6-meal/day plan which meant that she had to measure out her food portions (1-1.5 cups) before eating every 2½ hours.

At first her children laughed but later thought it was fun that she could eat seven times a day, and they joined her routine. When she exercised, she decreased her training intensity and bought a Polar® Heart Rate Monitor. She recorded her immediate heart rate (HR) and the average HR for each duration of training. After three months, Amy had lost 35 lbs. and 10 inches from her waist! Her husband, Ray, was jealous and he joined in her program. Together they lost a total of 90 pounds and have helped start ten of their friends in the RightSize weight loss program!

Return to Her Twenty-Something Shape

Mary started this program to focus on restoring her cardiovascular efficiency and reducing her cholesterol. Initially her weight was 220 lbs., and her waist size was 44 inches. Her initial cholesterol reading was high (220 mg/Dl), which is considered a high/risky threshold. Mary previously participated in a popular spin class four times a week but had no significant success in reducing her cholesterol or her waist size.

Her goal was to feel like she was twenty-something again! She then began following the RightSize PEN protocol of eating a measured portion size six times a day, exercising briefly before a meal, or eating only natural products. In six months she lost 40 lbs., six dress sizes (16 inches off her waist), and her cholesterol levels went from 220 to 150 mg/Dl. However, the greatest accomplishment was that Mary has maintained all these results for five years. She proudly proclaims, "Doc's PEN program helped me start a life where I always feel twenty-something." She also said that the additional teasing TIPS has even helped her sex life explode! (Her husband went from being addicted to his office work to being addicted to Mary's teasing.)

"Work Lunches" for Metabolism Acceleration

Pastor Bill always tried to get to the gym and eat the right foods, but his erratic schedule and work lunches had contributed to his overweight, inactive, sedentary state. He started using the Energy Surge exercise routine when he first awoke and later read devotions while riding the recumbent bicycle at the YMCA. He felt good about what he was doing and when he had meals at restaurants, he would limit his choices to using Portion size as his variable. He would often order a small hamburger without fries, which elevated his metabolism. He would always estimate how much of the plate's serving would fit in a cereal bowl.

Bill felt empowered by this and while he only needed to lose 20 lbs., he decreased his blood pressure from 160/80 to 125/75. After four more months, he was taken off his medicine for high cholesterol. Now when others ask about how to experience his success, he says to simply, "Honor God with your body."

Diabetes Cured!

Ten years ago Angie had become overweight and had developed Diabetes Type II. When she started the PEN program, she had high blood glucose and her HbA1c score was 12. (The HbA1c test gives an average of one's blood/glucose levels.) Nutrition was of great importance to Angie, but I also saw the need for the appropriate, low intensity exercise. She began the PEN program with a brisk walk 2-3 minutes before a meal and added low intensity cardiovascular exercise three times a week. Her program progressed as she added choices of Natural foods that met her needs for losing inches and blood glucose reductions.

Angie dropped 35 lbs. and her HbA1c has dropped from 12 to 8, which is a healthy, non-diabetic score. During the latter part of the first year, her primary care physician began reducing her medication for Type II Diabetes, and after two more years of a stable HbA1c and stable, permanent fat loss, her disease was pronounced cured by the RightSize program!

Fibromyalgia Cured!

Madi had suffered debilitating abrupt pain that made her fearful of any exercise. When she attended physical therapy sessions, the pain eruptions would start soon after she performed the short movement exercise routines like the pulley action exercise (up and down) on a wall rack. I taught her to use the Full Arc exercise that moved through her full range of motion for just a few minutes, twice a day. The Full Arc is where each joint is moved through the complete range of motion (full flexion to full extension) with light resistance. The frequency and intensity of her fibro eruptions both decreased, and then Madi started the PEN program to regain the attractive figure that she had before this disease limited her movement.

She said, "I was sedentary because excessive movement caused my fibromyalgia to erupt, and I would rather be heavy than in pain. Doc Willis designed a program to reduce the frequency and intensity of my pain (from fibromyalgia) and then I lost 40 lbs. which I have maintained for years!" "Thanks, Doc!" *(Madison R. from Austin, Texas)*

Beer Belly Traded for Six Pack

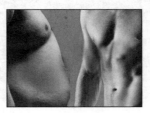

Mike played rugby for his university and never had a problem with a slow metabolism in college. However, after graduating, Mike quickly gained a beer belly, and his positions in club rugby changed from being an inside center (running back) to a flanker on the scrum because he was getting heavy and could not run as fast. After consulting with Doc, he realized that he was not eating often enough because he only ate two hamburgers, once a day.

He used PEN, particularly the Energy Surge for four months and lost 20 lbs., but his body became more dense. In a few more months, Mike had a six-pack to flash after the "old boys" had victory over a young college rugby team at a tournament.

Postpartum Pounds to Professional Model

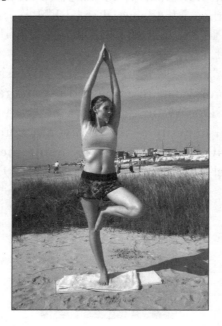

CJ lost her first child in delivery and soon became pregnant again. After delivery of her healthy, beautiful son, she felt hurt when she retained weight and people asked, "Are you pregnant again?" She began adding an Energy Surge quick walk to her daily routine. People often ask the question, "If you only use one of Doc's protocols, will it work?" CJ's answer is yes that the Energy Surge worked so well that she is now a professional model and can be seen in many of the fitness and stretching pictures!

Digest This

People have lost much weight with this easy, 3-option program that can be used at any time and at any event to lose weight. This can be used from dining with the President to eating Dutch pastries on a Caribbean beach!

2

Simple Adjustments

"My dilemma was that every gym I attended and every Weight Loss program I went to had the same 'one size fits all' type of program. Only Dr. Willis' program gave me the flexibility that I could put in MY program to lose 35 lbs. and keep the weight off for years. Thanks, Doc!" *(Amy B, Lakeway, Texas)*

Permanent change requires following five simple steps:
1) See or determine the need
2) Use the tools
3) Take action
4) Gain positive reinforcement
5) Progress to higher goals

First, you have **determined your need** for a change since you have purchased this book; congratulations, you have already taken the first step. Next you should schedule a physical exam with your Primary Care Physician (PCP). Tell your PCP you are intent on starting a holistic weight loss program including Portion control while eating five meals a day + Energy Surge exercise + Natural Nutrition (PEN), and you would like a full blood test including lipid profile, HbA1c (mean glucose), and a thyroid panel.

Body Summation

It is important to include your doctor, have baseline testing, and be aware of any physical limitations your doctor may alert you of. During this examination, ask if your doctor's nurse or assistant can take all the girth measurements or have a friend or relative help you. (Neck, shoulders, upper arm [widest], wrist, chest, waist, hips [widest], upper thigh [widest], calf, and ankle) in inches. Record these measurements by filling out the Body Summation form on page 159, (making copies of it to use in subsequent months.)

The Body Summation is an ideal barometer for measuring change in weight loss rather than just your BMI. If your BMI is greater than 30 then you are at risk, but it takes a significant change to move the BMI; whereas, the Body Summation shows reduction of fat, which is the lightest substance in our human bodies (lighter than water). It is also a risk factor if a person's waistline is more than half of their height. So while we're reducing the waistline, let's also measure victorious reductions in the neck, hips, thighs, etc.

Seeing your progress is important, so you will need to fill out the Body Summation form once a month for your feedback. Hide your bathroom scale from daily use! To complete the Body Summation form, all you will need is a cloth tape measure and a scale to measure weight once a month.

We're all different, so there is not a "good or bad" Body Summation, but we all can have a *good change* in our score, no matter where we start! Your first goal should be to achieve a 5% reduction in your Body Summation. Then future, long term goals can be set for reducing the total Body Summation score more if appropriate.

Explosive changes will also require methodical, incremental steps to ensure their permanency. The FDA and CDC suggest a slow loss of 2-5 lbs. per month, which should reinforce the fact that you need not work too hard.

You will receive feedback from friends and family when your dress size changes or there is a visibility of abdominal muscles, but it's more important to raise your metabolism and keep it there. Instead of pounds you need to stay focused on the Body Summation score and your goal to RightSize your physique. Your Body Summation will show your true victory, because it takes many small changes to whittle a large, rough stump of wood into a trim, beautiful, sculpture!

Second, **use the tools** and remember that for the first week or more you should plan in advance specifically which strategy you will use for each dining event. For example, Natural for meal #1 (fruit and whole oats with milk), Exercise before eating #2 (AdvoCare nutrition bar), Portion size for a business lunch #3 (steak and veggies), Natural for your afternoon snack #4 (an apple), and Exercise with your family or friends right before your final meal #5 like soup. Remember, "Forecast your food." Also stop all food from passing your lips three hours before bed so that you have a nightly fasting for full digestion of what you have eaten during the day.

Third, **take action**—now is the time to start taking action and use PEN in one of your dining events today. Plan to start an easy exercise routine to include just ten minutes a few times a week. For example, have a Cardio Monday and Wednesday, ten stretching exercises once a week, and "Body Resistance" once a week. PEN is what will help you lose weight and gain your RightSize, but these additional exercise sessions will help retain or increase bone mass density, muscle tone, and cardiovascular health.

Fourth, you need accountability and **positive reinforcement** with feedback and encouragement for your successes and challenges. It is important to involve your friends and family for local support. When you reach a goal, who will you brag to? If you have a pessimist in your life, do not choose that person. Shake off the doubters and choose to see your success through a positive friend's eyes. Choose a person who is always uplifting.

Who will be your accountability partner? If it is a family member, then test the water to see exactly what they say when you announce that you are starting a "wellness program that will help me lose weight." What is their first reaction? Write it down and perhaps share that with your consultant at the www.DocWillis.org website for support and accountability (more about the website later).

Fifth, we need to have continual baby steps to **progress to higher, different goals**. For example, as you read in the testimonies, one man went from coat size 46 to size 38 and lost four inches in his waist with a healthy reduction of his BMI. Then he changed his goals to be more athletically focused for bicycle spring racing!

DIGEST THIS

You have seen the need to improve your wellness, weight, and health. The simple, flexible tools are laid out in this book. After finishing this chapter, why not move on to increase your heart rate? Then gain positive reinforcement from a friend or family member and see how to start with just one step to reach even higher goals!

3

Why Other Programs Fail

"I had tried every diet and it seemed like I had been on a diet most every year from age 22 to 42. It wasn't until I started Doc's easy program that I found success and inspiration to keep losing! I've have been on my RightSize program for two years, and I still feel better every day!" *(Rachel Ray, Dallas, Texas)*

Fad diets often work for a short period, but they have limitations and are not flexible enough for all situations. Sixty percent of the people in developed countries are overweight because of sedentary behavior, abundant chemical additives/preservatives in the food, and high emotional stress, (compared to people living in the early 1800s). The key reasons why fad diets and aggressive exercise programs fail over time is that while they shock the body into change, it takes more than just a lowering of calories to regain or obtain the RightSize for a lifetime. It takes conscious efforts to raise one's metabolism at every chance.

Counting calories or food points may work for a while, but it does nothing to accelerate your metabolism. Many diet programs that cut calories actually lower one's metabolism. That is why these programs have limited success in changing the body's shape. How effective are counting points when one attends a catered business luncheon, or what variability does the Atkins diet have for Christmas or birthday parties? Programs like Weight Watchers and Jenny Craig work because they combine education, food products, and peer support. However, their programs have been around for decades and our planet is till obese.

I say "Eat cake and lose weight," and with my program you will accelerate your metabolism in any circumstance! The program that you will start (with tutelage from me) will allow flexibility for all occasions. It is easy and admirable to start a weight loss program, but it is hard to finish a plan unless the protocol is easy! Here are the most common problems in weight loss that my program will help you avoid.

Avoid Failure

Thousands of people start exercise training, but they drop out from lack of success. How many people who started going to a gym as a New Year's goal last January are still exercising? Here are the most common reasons why.

Training too hard causes delayed muscle soreness, which is the underlying factor that impairs most new exercise regimes. This soreness is the inflammation from micro trauma to the skeletal muscle fibers. The concept of "No pain no gain" is good in body building, but for weight loss it is counterproductive. The most common cause for discontinuing exercise is pain.

Pain can be avoided by training at a lower level rather than too high of a one, and cooling down for five minutes after the exercise. For example if your cardio exercise was on a Lifecycle, after you have completed the 20+ minutes at your target heart rate, then take the intensity to level 0 and just pedal easily for five minutes. Then perform four or more leg/ankle stretches (See chapter 12). The cool down plus stretching will reabsorb the lactic acid, which is generated through the muscular contractions, and this will prevent muscle soreness the second day.

Lack of social interaction is another common cause of dropping out of an exercise program. One benefit of going to a gym or health club is that you can attend with friends or make new friends there. After you read this book, you can be adopted into our mentorship program with veterans who will support your success. (This is the program membership at www.DocWillis.org.) If you train at a gym, take the book with you and introduce yourself to someone also exercising. Ask how long they have been going there and then ask what days they schedule for training next week. It helps to have people who know you, and the chat may be a more enjoyable distraction that just reading a book, although reading can help pass the time. One of our pastors did his daily Bible reading on an elliptical four mornings a week. My sweetie would rather perform a brisk walk on the beach, which is also spiritually nourishing for her, and my favorite exercise is bicycling with the ocean breezes blowing. Experiment to see what works the best for you.

Lack of reinforcement is another reason for not continuing an exercise regime. For this reason, we have the Body Summation table that will give you measurable feedback each month to reinforce your continued, accelerated success. For this evaluation you need to choose an optimistic person who will help with measurements and encourage you through this journey. This person could be a positive, resourceful friend, or you can have this data collected at your doctor's office. Having a 20 point reduction in your first month will be a rewarding and encouraging outcome. Let's say "Can do!" At the same time, realize that your goals must be logical and appropriate. For example, how long did it take to gain 20 extra pounds of belly fat? Only allocating four weeks to permanently lose that weight may be unrealistic.

The barriers to change can also include "reward values." If it is more appealing to have a tangible first step such as "fit into my skinny jeans," then use that as a higher priority for reinforcement. The main outcome will still become a healthier, RightSize lifestyle. Champion weight loss victors on Doc's team could also be there to help reinforce your work. They have used his program for explosive weight loss, and they can coach you too.

Procrastination, de-prioritization, misplaced gratification, and rationalizations also deter the most sincere, meaningful starts. Before each meal you must consciously decide if you will use Portion size, Exercise, or Natural nutrition to accelerate your metabolism. Remember to do the "Food forecast" each day. Gratification should come through changes in your Body Summation Score. If you need to hear feedback and praise for your efforts, tell your partner, spouse, or clinician that you need to hear this.

You have started on the best pathway to RightSize your body with the purchase of this book. Including TIPS (that will be discussed later in the book) into your daily lifestyle will ensure that you automatically "change up" your activity schedule and exercise routine to reach your physical goals. TIPS include using different 2-3 minute exercises to elevate your HR into the Aerobic Threshold. The right quick exercise or eating will tease the body into a higher metabolic rate, and then regular cardio exercise will be even more effective to reduce weight, volume, and inches.

DIGEST THIS

Training too hard and trying to progress too fast can lead to program failure. The RightSize program will let you use different options, which is different from many programs that have too stringent restrictions for long term success.

4

Easy, Natural, Permanent Change

"I felt ugly because I was always gaining weight, and never consistently weighing less, even though I was on at least two diets per year. Doc helped me make the change that I enjoyed seeing myself having a smaller Summation Body count each month, and now I am a big, beautiful, FIRM woman!" *(Angela P. Laredo, Texas)*

Let's more fully look into the three simple steps to creating your customized, flexible, unique formula that I have labelled **PEN**. To recap, they are:

• **P**ortion Size—Eat every 2-3 hours with a limited amount (1.5 cups) that will be metabolized in two hours. (This is what makes body builders so lean before a contest.) Do this with six meals per day.

• **E**nergy Surge (elevated heart rate for 2-3 minutes before you even get out of bed in the morning and ideally before every meal.) This is flexible but important to complete at least three times a day.

• **N**atural Foods are the choice foods to eat at least three times a day (unprocessed foods as eaten 100 years ago).

This is the PEN formula: Portion size, Energy Surge

21

Exercise, or Nutrition. You will use one of these three components before each meal to raise your metabolism and enjoy the most efficient, complete digestion of your food.

Portion Size

The Portion Size component of this formula came from when I was a bodybuilder and prepared for physique pictures. **The rule is to eat foods that do not exceed a soup bowl serving (1.5 cups) five to six times a day.** Since our goal is to RightSize, this technique can be used in any setting. For example, Ray and Rachel would always perform their "children exchange" at McDonalds. Rachel felt awkward when she tried to buy diet foods there, when the Big Mac was what she craved. After starting her RightSize program, she guessed that she could join her daughter in eating a "Happy Meal" with its four chicken sticks.

She took a Happy Meal home and sure enough it all fit into a 1½ measuring cup. The Happy Meal gave her a protein, carbs, and fruit. She often would tell the children later that they inspired her weight loss of 30 lbs. When her children grew to be teenagers, they would remember and brag that "all meals are happy when we are happy." Now Rachel has returned to equestrian competition (that she first started as a college student at Texas State University), and she often eats a good protein bar like a Cliff Builder's Bar (20 g protein) every few hours when she is working with her horse.

Energy Surge

Remember, exercise does not have to be long durations in the gym but rather fun, quick bouts like the kids do. Let's mimic the activity pattern that we had when we were kids with high metabolic rates. Participating in short, high-energy, bouts of exercise (2-3 minute Energy Surge) a few times a day will make a tremendous difference in your physique but also your bone mass density, cardiovascular health, etc. More will be described in the next chapter and next section. (Get approval from your physician first for safety.)

Using the Energy Surge exercise before eating is ideal for occasions when a meal cannot be controlled with natural nutrition or portion size. When Amy had to attend events that she organized for her church, she felt obligated to share the food. Before such an event, she would perform a brisk walk/jog around the church to get her heart rate over 135 (which was 75% of her max heart rate at age 41). The Aerobic Threshold will be discussed in greater detail later, but use this description to understand how and why this target heart rate is important. If you were running away from a bear the fastest your heart would beat would equal 220 - your age. For a 41 year old that would be 179 beats/minute. The aerobic threshold is 75% of that max and approximately 134 beats/minute is when you body consumes the most oxygen and uses fat as the primary fuel!

She kept walking at this rate for just three minutes, which was enough to elevate her basal metabolic rate but not long enough to start excessive sweating. She'd then rejoin her congregation for the luncheon. Pretty soon a few of the youth joined her, and her church began a RightSize Formula program for the community, proclaiming the verses in 1 Cor. 6:19-20 as God's Word on this effort! You can see more examples and information to create your own perfect, Energy Surge exercise in chapters 6 and 13.

Natural Foods

All Natural Foods is a strong component in the PEN formula because research has shown that excessive chemicals slow our metabolism. While Organic Foods are ideal, consumption of more readily available and less expensive grocery products is equally beneficial in this component. This takes planning and forethought, but this protocol can be the most beneficial. It is similar to the Raw Diet craze, but it allows food to be cooked. Unlike the Atkins Diet, it does allow consumption of natural (unprocessed) carbohydrates that are needed for optimal nutrition.

Here is a great example. For lunch Reneé, an RN, would bring her lunch, which included delicious grilled fish, fresh green beans, a small sweet potato, and homemade salsa (fresh tomatoes, red onion, peppers, cilantro, etc.).

Reneé ate only natural foods until she was full, and she often had leftovers. She did not consume anything processed so she did not eat bread or use Ranch dressing or any commercially prepared sauces. Eating a natural food lunch left her satisfied. Remember that when consuming only natural foods, your beverages must also be natural such as water, squeezed juice, or home brewed tea leaves.

An important part of PEN is that we encourage you to "Forecast your food!" Keeping a food diary for the first two weeks will help you plan and benefit from your choices. Buy a small notebook and write down everything that passes your lips for the first week or so. (See "Let's Get Real," Chapter 9.)

Beverages

The beverages you choose to consume are important in

your RightSize Formula. All beverages are good (in moderation), but recent research has surprisingly shown that over-consumption of diet drinks can actually be associated with weight gain. A scholar on weight loss, Dr. Ferreira, along with his colleagues, accomplished an epidemiological study in September 2014, which showed the "paradoxical association between low-calorie beverages and weight gain." Their research explained why low-calorie drinks actually increase appetite. These drinks increase the appetite for carbohydrates while reducing metabolism, which causes a greater portion of foods consumed to be stored as fat!

The bottom line is that drinks with sugar substitutes should be avoided. However, beverages containing natural sweetening such as "Throw Back Mountain Dew" or "TING" (delicious carbonated grapefruit juice from the Caribbean that is available in HEB, Whole Foods, and Kroger stores) would be more desirable than drinks sweetened with high fructose corn syrup, an ingredient included in almost all processed sweet drinks and foods. Obviously sugars are to be avoided for people with diabetes mellitus, but this is also where our nutritionist could help you make enjoyable, smart beverage choices. For people without diabetes, the rule is to overall pick sugar instead of diet drinks to lose weight!

Drinking wine and alcohol will be described in detail in chapter 9, but such beverages have been shown to be beneficial (in moderation) to one's health. Be careful because calories from beer and alcohol are "empty" in the direct benefits one gains, because alcohol is digested differently than other foods.

Normally the carbohydrates, fats, and proteins are broken down in the gastrointestinal (GI) system, but alcohol triggers the response as a toxin would. Since it is in a liquid form, it passes through the GI system rapidly, and the small intestine absorbs it quickly to eliminate the ethanol from the system. This causes its fast absorption into the blood that quickly reaches the brain. When alcohol reaches the liver for elimination, only small amounts are processed immediately. This is an example of how drinking just one glass of wine or one bottle of beer will not impair weight loss goals, but drinking large volumes will.

Additionally alcohol is a diuretic and it will carry away water that is needed for digestion, causing a reduced metabolic rate and increased dehydration. This causes one to lose important minerals such as potassium and calcium. This book includes significant research that proves the efficacy of these protocols. For example, a study of 19,220 women over age 39 by Dr. Lu Wang (2010) and colleagues, showed that consuming one drink every day did not have a negative effect on their weight over the span of 13 years. However, if one saves up the daily drinks in order to consume seven drinks on a Saturday night, then it will lead to weight gain and decreased metabolism. Drinking one glass of wine every evening would actually be far better for weight loss than drinking one diet soda a day.

DIGEST THIS

The **PEN** program starts with using one or more of three methods: **P**ortion Control: eating 1.5 cups 6 times per day) that will be metabolized in a two hours, **E**nergy Surge exercise to elevate your heart rate for just a few minutes, eating **N**atural Nutrition of organic, unprocessed foods. Use any of the three to boost your energy level to burn more fat as fuel.

5

Where Are You Now?

"I have dieted and exercised for years but with no prolonged success. I went from uninspired and couch
potato to active, healthy, and fit. This was because of
Doc's amazingly simple, easy, and enjoyable program!"
*(Jim S. from Austin, Texas, lost 31 lbs. in two months
and has kept it off.)*

Chemicals in Our Food

We have an overweight epidemic caused by excessive,
chemical additives in packaged, processed food. How many
chemicals are you eating today? Most commercial food products include chemicals. The bottom line is why is it good for
you to eat something you have never seen? A famous nutritionist says "eat only things that come from the earth!" Even
an "All Natural" product of nuts and fruit product pictured on
the next page includes sulfur dioxides and other preservatives.

Our bodies were not made to consume the often toxic
chemicals included in commercially produced, packaged food
products. Additives are commonly included in popular commercially manufactured foods, which cause morbidity and
mortality. The following is a list of chemicals for "healthy
nuts."

Ingredients:
PEANUTS (ROASTED IN PEANUT
OIL), BANANA CHIPS (COCONUT
OIL), SUGAR, BANANA
FLAVORING, RAISINS,
SUNFLOWER KERNELS, DATES
WITH OAT FLOWER
COATINGALMONDS,
APPRICOTS, SULPHUR IODIDE
USED FOR FRESHNESS

Arsenic: This is a carcinogenic substance that has been linked to cancer of the lungs, kidney, and bladder. Arsenic is often found in grape and apple juice.

Aspartame (Artificial Sweetener): Research has shown that diet sodas actually slow down the metabolism and increase carbohydrate cravings, leading to gain weight. There are numerous diseases that are caused, enhanced, or aggravated by these chemicals. Aspartame is carcinogenic and has been clearly associated with brain tumors and lymphoma. It also contributes to pathologies such as migraine headaches, diabetes, multiple sclerosis, Parkinson's, Alzheimer's, fibromyalgia, and other diseases. This is found in most diet sodas. The bottom line is that sugar from natural sugar cane in small doses will actually raise your metabolism!

Bisphenol A (BPA) and Phthalates: BPA has been linked to abnormally accelerated pubescent development in children. These are additives in plastics that bind to food products heated in the microwave ovens. If you use a microwave, transfer the food to a glass dish before heating. Microwave action frees the BPA, which then attach to the food particles.

Carnauba Wax: Used for consistency in chewing gum and can cause cancer and oral tumors.

Carmel Food Coloring (4-Mel): This additive has been proven to be carcinogenic. In a test completed by *Consumer Reports* (2013), the levels of the additives of Pepsi One and Malta Goya purchased were >29 micrograms, which are higher than the maximum allowed without caution labels in California. When sold in California these drinks should have a readable label that states, "possibly carcinogenic to humans," similar to the labels required on cigarettes. The 4-Mel chemical is found in drinks like Pepsi One and even Pop-Tarts.

High Fructose Corn Syrup (HFC): Another manufactured sweetener that has been added to an abundant number of food products. It is actually one of the highest sources of calories in commercial food, but these are wasted calories because they burn quickly and easily with limited benefit other than quick transition into blood sugar and body fat. It has been shown to also raise the LDL—bad cholesterol—and there are few commercially processed foods that do not have HFC. It is surprisingly found in breads baked in grocery stores (plus commercial breads), salad dressings, cereal, and canned vegetables. If you eat at a restaurant that does not have a pastry chef, you are probably consuming packaged commercial foods with HFC.

Monosodium Glutamate (MSG): Used to enhance the flavor in protein-rich foods like fish, meats, and milk. This is commonly used in commercial, restaurant-prepared foods where you are not able to see the ingredient labels. MSG can cause migraine headaches, chronic inflammation, liver cancer, central obesity, type II diabetes, and fatty liver disease. The fatty liver disease can also lead to cirrhosis. We think of soup as a healthy food that we feed family members who are ill, but we need to read the labels. MSG is even included in Campbell's Minestrone soup.

Potassium Bromate: A substance shown to cause cancer in animal studies, and this is found in commercial bread products.

Red and Yellow Dyes (Red-40, Tartazine, Azo Dye, and Sunset Yellow: These dyes are banned in foods produced in the UK, the Netherlands, and Sweden; however, these chemicals are still in our children's macaroni & cheese. During the last 50 years, use of these toxins increased 500%. They cause damage to the immune system and errors in cell replication. This means the children who eat these toxins may have abnormal chromosome replication patterns. There are published hypotheses stating that food dyes could be causing the increase incidence of ADHD.

Refined Vegetable Oils: These include soybean oil, safflower oil, canola oil, and peanut oil. These products can cause headaches and digestive disorders and are linked to heart disease and cancer. Such oils are common in packaged snack foods from animal crackers to chocolate covered peanuts.

Sodium Benzoate: This is used as a preservative in salad dressing and carbonated beverages, and it is a known carcinogen and may cause damage DNA. This would yield damaged cell structures from that point on. Let's pick one: avoid eating a product or possible cell damage forever?

Sodium Nitrate or Nitrite: Packaged proteins are often treated with this toxic chemical in products such as lunch meat, hotdogs, corned beef, smoked fish, etc. This is also a highly carcinogenic chemical. Our bodies were not made to deal with ingesting such artificial lab chemicals. In response to these chemicals, our bodies start producing excessive, useless cells. When no longer controlled, cell production occurs, and it can become a tumor. These chemicals have been shown to cause liver and pancreas disease and cancer.

Why are we still suffering with products that cause disease? The United States Food and Drug Administration (FDA) tried to ban use of sodium nitrite in the 1970s, but political lobbyists controlled the politicians who stopped funding of this investigation.

Sodium Phosphate: Has been shown to cause serious kidney damage in some people including permanent renal damage requiring dialysis. This chemical also causes headaches and is commonly found in cheeses, salad dressings, packaged snack or breakfast foods, and non-dairy creamers.

Sodium Sulfite: Many people are sensitive to sulfites, which could make this additive an immediately life threatening toxin. It can also cause celiac disease. This additive is common in snack foods such as Chex mix, raisins, red wines, and balsamic vinegar.

Sucralose (Splenda®): Another artificial sweetener that has been shown to cause leukemia in mice that were exposed to it from before birth. Further studies have shown that sucralose causes DNA damage in mice and causes cancer. Sucralose is contained in packaged sweets and many dairy products. This includes low-fat flavored milk, light yogurt, low-fat coffee creamer, cereal bars, light ice cream, licorice, popsicles, canned fruit, factory baked goods (muffins), light tea, light maple syrup, jams, and jellies.

Sulfur Dioxide: This is a toxic substance prohibited by the FDA in raw fruits and vegetables because it causes bronchial disease and accelerated adverse reactions for people suffering from asthma, hypotension (low blood pressure), emphysema, or cardiovascular disease. This is found in beer, soft drinks, dried fruit, juices, cordials, wine, vinegar, and potato products.

Tertiary Butylhydroquinone (TBHQ): A common food additive/preservative that seems innocent but consuming just over one gram can cause delirium, nausea, tinnitus (ringing in the ears), and vomiting. It has also been suggested that it contributes to ADHD in children. It is also suggested that it may be responsible for affecting estrogen levels in women. This is found in flour-based, packaged food such as breakfast muffins.

Trans Fats (Partially hydrogenated vegetable oils): Such fats are still found in crackers, icing, cooking oils (for frying foods), margarine, and microwave popcorn. This is true even though trans-fats are directly linked with higher occurrence of cardiovascular heart disease and stroke.

Let's look at a specific example of Blueberry Pop-Tarts (which used to be one of my favorite movie snacks). In reading this expanded label above, one can see 15 chemical additives that have been shown to cause or contribute to illness, disease, and cancer. The chemicals are not digestible, and this contributes to the overweight epidemic. Such foods cannot be included in the Natural nutrition category for

INGREDIENTS: ENRICHED FLOUR (WHEAT FLOUR, NIACIN, REDUCED IRON, VITAMIN B_1 [THIAMIN MONONITRATE], VITAMIN B_2 [RIBOFLAVIN], FOLIC ACID), CORN SYRUP, HIGH FRUCTOSE CORN SYRUP, DEXTROSE, SOYBEAN AND PALM OIL (WITH TBHQ FOR FRESHNESS). SUGAR, CRACKER MEAL, CONTAINS TWO PERCENT OR LESS OF WHEAT STARCH, SALT, DRIED BLUEBERRIES, DRIED GRAPES, DRIED APPLES, LEAVENING (BAKING SODA, SODIUM ACID PYROPHOSPHATE, MONOCALCIUM PHOSPHATE), CITRIC ACID, MILLED CORN, GELATIN, SOYBEAN OIL, MODIFIED CORN STARCH, MODIFIED WHEAT STARCH, SOY LECITHIN, XANTHAN GUM, CARAMEL COLOR, RED 40, VITAMIN A PALMITATE, NIACINAMIDE, REDUCED IRON, NATURAL AND ARTIFICIAL FLAVOR, BLUE 2, BLUE 1, VITAMIN B_6 (PYRIDOXINE HYDROCHLORIDE), COLOR ADDED, TURMERIC EXTRACT, VITAMIN B_2 (RIBOFLAVIN), VITAMIN B_1 (THIAMIN HYDROCHLORIDE).
CONTAINS WHEAT AND SOY INGREDIENTS.

weight loss. A good rule of thumb is that if a food product has more than five ingredients, then you need to examine the label more closely or choose another product. The bottom line should be that if you cannot hold a substance in your hand (i.e. TBHQ) then it should not be eaten!

CLIFF Builder's protein bars have lots of ingredients but a much healthier label than Pop-Tarts:

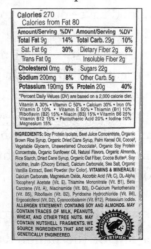

Calories 270
Calories from Fat 80

Amount/Serving	%DV*	Amount/Serving	%DV*
Total Fat 9g	14%	Total Carb. 29g	10%
Sat. Fat 6g	30%	Dietary Fiber 2g	8%
Trans Fat 0g		Insoluble Fiber 2g	
Cholesterol 0mg	0%	Sugars 22g	
Sodium 200mg	8%	Other Carb. 5g	
Potassium 190mg	5%	Protein 20g	40%

*Percent Daily Values (DV) are based on a 2,000 calorie diet.

Vitamin A 30% • Vitamin C 50% • Calcium 30% • Iron 0%
Vitamin D 10% • Vitamin E 50% • Vitamin (B1) 10%
Riboflavin (B2) 15% • Niacin (B3) 15% • Vitamin B6 25%
Vitamin B12 15% • Pantothenic Acid 20% • Iodine 10%
Magnesium 15%

INGREDIENTS: Soy Protein Isolate, Beet Juice Concentrate, Organic Brown Rice Syrup, Organic Dried Cane Syrup, Palm Kernel Oil, Cocoa², Vegetable Glycerine, Unsweetened Chocolate², Organic Soy Protein Concentrate, Organic Sunflower Oil, Natural Flavors, Organic Almonds, Rice Starch, Dried Cane Syrup, Organic Oat Fiber, Cocoa Butter², Soy Lecithin, Inulin (Chicory Extract), Calcium Carbonate, Sea Salt, Organic Vanilla Extract, Beet Powder (for Color). VITAMINS & MINERALS: Calcium Carbonate, Magnesium Oxide, Ascorbic Acid (Vit. C), DL-Alpha Tocopheryl Acetate (Vit. E), Thiamine Mononitrate (Vit. B1), Beta Carotene (Vit. A), Niacinamide (Vit. B3), D-Calcium Pantothenate (Vit. B5), Riboflavin (Vit. B2), Pyridoxine Hydrochloride (Vit. B6), Ergocalciferol (Vit. D2), Cyanocobalamin (Vit. B12), Potassium Iodide. ALLERGEN STATEMENT: CONTAINS SOY AND ALMONDS. MAY CONTAIN TRACES OF MILK, PEANUTS, WHEAT, AND OTHER TREE NUTS. MAY CONTAIN NUTSHELL FRAGMENTS. WE SOURCE INGREDIENTS THAT ARE NOT GENETICALLY ENGINEERED.

However, the Lara Bars win the race in simple, chemical free, healthy snacks! (See below for list of ingredients.)

LARABAR™
INGREDIENTS: DATES, CASHEWS, ALMONDS, RAISINS, CINNAMON, GINGER, ALLSPICE, VANILLA EXTRACT

Listen to Your Body!

Give your body tastes of natural and/or organic foods to see and feel the difference. When eating a meal served at a restaurant that makes you feel bloated, overly full, or causes stomach muscle discomfort, write it down. Then on a following day at the same time, eat only natural foods of the same volume and see how your stomach reacts differently. What and how much processed food have you been consuming?

Now is the time for readers to start a Food Log for your first week in the program. Use a small notebook and write down everything you eat and drink. Or you can go to our website and download the handy Food Log app. Try to estimate portions (1 cup of Cheerios cereal with 1/2 cup of 2% milk). This will take a little effort but it helps you see where you are starting. This will give you insight as to where PEN will help you the most.

Let's Write Your Victory

You have read a few of the hundreds of success stories and now let's start writing your story of success. Know that you will be a victor not a victim as you regain your RightSize. Read these questions, and make a check mark beside the experiences you have had. Also write a note if you remember something significant that you experienced. Beyond just reading, start participating in your success.

• Have you been eating lots of chemicals in processed foods?

• When was the last time you ate only natural foods for one full day?

• Was there an event in your life that triggered a change in weight or body size?

• Have you always been a little heavy?

• Did you start gaining weight after delivery of a child?

• Did you start gaining weight after an orthopedic injury or surgery? (Some former college athletes have developed arthritis, which keeps them from training, but using RightSize for their weight has also improved their joint function.)

• Did you start gaining weight after as an emotional event such as a divorce or when you lost your job? (Emotional traumas have many results, but having confidence in your body image helps your overall self-image.)

• Has depression reduced your activity level? (Depression is a clinical disease that we should not be ashamed of, and it can be treated with the right exercise to balance the serotonin levels.)

• Are you are on anti-depressant medication and has this clearly caused you to gain weight? Then talk to your doctor and do not just stop taking the prescribed medication. Your physician may choose another medication. Be sure to tell your doctor that you are starting the PEN program with proven exercise protocols. The right prescribed exercise has been shown to clearly reduce depression. Exercise compliments traditional treatments, and we will talk about that in Section 3.

• Do you have stress at the office and are without time for the gym each day? (Stress causes secretion of cortisol, which is the stress hormone, and this increases our appetite. Have a supply of stress snacks on hand. You can also sprint up a few flights of stairs or do 50 jumping jacks if possible.)

• Do you gain weight because you are always hungry? (Consumption of quick carbohydrates, like a bag of chips, actually makes your body want more cheap quality carbs. We will help you plan five quality "Fuel Up" meals. (You can read about this in chapter 7.) If you can dedicate 2-3 minutes, twice a day, and ingest Natural foods three times a day, you will have less hunger and your new RightSize!

• Are you happiest when eating ice cream or chips while watching TV? (You can eat organic ice cream in a way that elevates your metabolism when you RightSize the portion and timing.)

• Has your life recently changed? Have the children started school, have they gone off to college, or have you retired? (Good news! These are significant differences that can actually be used to help improve your fitness and this has been done many times. See chapter 5.)

• Are you short on sleep and are you too tired to exercise? (While exercise has been clinically tested to help to improve sleep patterns, it is sometimes hard to start the right way.

Food choices when in a sleep deprivation cycle make the disorder worse. Look in Chapter 13 to learn more about this.)

• Has dieting made you gain weight over time? (This is common for many people and that is why you're reading this book. Say it out loud, "I will make the change *without* a diet!" Dietary changes are only one leg of a three-legged stool, and sometimes that leg needs to have more freedom. The change can happen through exercise/energy-level or through eating Natural foods. RightSize is the first to make all options possible for a faster, easier outcome.)

• When you reached a significant age (40 or 50) did your metabolism just fall off the charts? (Hormonal changes that happen as we age can be changed with the right exercise and the right fuel or natural foods that restore hormone levels and higher metabolism.)

• Have you been diagnosed with low, hypothyroid secretions? (This affects over 4% of the population and can be treated both clinically and with complementary natural methods. Take your doctor's advice and why not try all options to see what is effective for you?)

• Are you weaker than ever before? (When you are weak with reduced activity, it causes muscle atrophy [muscle shrinkage], and this is a difficult spiral to overcome. After you read this chapter, go immediately to chapter 6 and do one of the 2-3 minute Energy Surge exercises. You just started the change for a lifetime! Good job!)

• Do you gain weight when you try to quit smoking? (Stopping smoking is the best thing you can do for your life and wellness, but initially it also causes metabolism slow down and an increase in carbohydrate cravings. Use a gradual withdrawal program with specific exercises described in chapter 6 to RightSize while stopping the cause of 1,000 different diseases!)

• What else has caused you to gain weight? (You know yourself the best and when you have regained your RightSize, there could be many people who would benefit from your experience! Please write this down because I am interested in featuring you in the next book on RightSize Success!)

DIGEST THIS

Our country has become the most overweight nation on the planet because we have the largest use of preservative, stabilizers, and other processed chemical additives in our food than any other country. Our body does not know how to digest these chemicals, and processing them through the liver has been shown to slow the metabolism. This is why drinking diet sodas with aspartame has been shown to gain weight.

SECTION II

Activate Your Energy Surge

6

Ignite Your Metabolism

"I hated aerobics college PE course. It was a defeating experience because I did not know how to enjoy my movement. Doc Willis helped me find the movement that I enjoy, which can yield an elevated heart rate for fat consumption!" *(Thaise E, Kilgore, Texas)*

A quick 3-minute Energy Surge exercise right before you eat will increase your metabolism and help you burn more fat. The following are 25 easy example exercises that won't make you sweat but will get your heart rate (HR) to 75% of your maximum. Please consult your physician first and let them brag on your success later. Doctors will warn you that if you get lightheaded or dizzy after such an exercise bout, then you need to stop because you may have other health care needs that must be addressed.

Energy Surge

These easy exercises are in alphabetical order but try them all over the next few weeks to see which ones challenge you and become your favorites to accelerate your metabolism. Each exercise should be challenging enough to raise your heart rate (HR) to 75% of your maximum. [To calculate:

(220-age) x .75 = target HR] If your heart rate is not this elevated, then you can use these exercises in regular training, but they do not count as your intense pre-meal exercise.

1) **Arm Spins**: Extend both arms while standing on a firm surface (not carpet). At first swing as fast as you can from side to side. Then swing your arms while you pick up one foot and spin. Perform 100 for the right duration.

2) **Bed Drapes** are a unique home pre-meal exercise that target your abdominal muscles. Stand with your back to the bed and sit with your hips on the edge of the bed. Recline with your back on the bed and your hands overhead. Now let your legs drape over the edge of the bed and briskly raise your feet to the ceiling.

3) **Brain Busters**

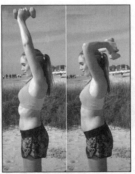

These can be performed with two full 16 oz. cans or bottles of liquid. Holding the cans, sit in the chair and simply touch your fingers to your ears and then extend the can until your arms are straight. Now repeat the exercise, quickly for 100 times to get an elevated heart rate and Energy Surge!

4) **Board Hinge**: Stand and hold your hands over your head. While holding your body stiff as a plank, quickly bend

at your waist down to touch your toes. Then quickly return to the upright position 20 times. If you can do more, then keep adding five more repetitions until you are moving for 2-3 continual minutes.

5) **Bounce a Basketball** as fast as you can with two hands 100 times. Bounce from the ground to your chest.

6) **Clock Swings**: Pick up the basketball and quickly swing from a 2 o'clock position to 7 o'clock position 20 times. Then swing from 5 o'clock to 11 o'clock another 20 times. Is your heart rate elevated? If not, then do it all two times again but faster.

7) **Crunches** are the classic abdominal maneuver where you lay on your back and bring your knees slightly toward your head and your shoulders towards your waist. (Don't lift your neck!) Pull your body together and hold for a count of 180 seconds.

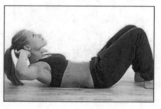

8) **Curls**

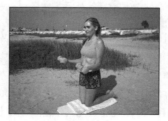

Curls can be accomplished with soup cans or light dumb-bells (DB). Simply curl as many times as you can with your palms up, and as many times as you can, holding the can upright like a hammer.

9) **Downward Facing Dog**

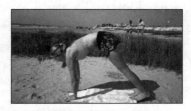

Start by laying prone (tummy down) and then moving to hands and knees touching the floor (doggie). Then step onto your feet and walk your feet closer to your hands and back down. Now go from the flat, prone position to the flexed "dog" position 20 times.

10) **Forward Lunge:**

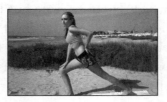

With your body in the upright position, simply take a long step out and let one knee bend towards the ground. For the Energy Surge, complete a brisk 12 lunges in 30 seconds. To make this an effective exercise, perform 24 for each leg and the total duration it takes to step forward to lunge and return should be a slow 30 seconds.

11) **Glute Bridge:** Lay on your back with your face to the ceiling (supine) and walk your heels back to elevate your hips. Hold this for three minutes or you can include up and down motions to prolong your duration for 3 minutes.

12) **Jumping Jacks:** Clap your hands above your head followed by slapping the side of your thighs. Two to three minutes is your goal at 75% of your max HR.

13) **Pedal Upside Down:** This was used by one of our victors. She lay on her back and moved her feet as if she were riding a bicycle upside down. Again this must elevate your HR and be challenging to count as a pre-meal exercise.

14) **Pushups:**

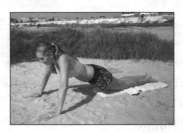

Pushups are an old school favorite but holding your body in a solid plank while you lower your chest to the ground activates many muscles as stabilizers as well. Women start with your knees on the ground. CJ can out push most people. Two to three minutes of pushups will be a lot for great success.

15) **Push Ups with Single Leg Raise:** Do the pushup and then raise one leg making this a tripod pose. After obtaining the pose, then perform pushups and alternate between legs for three minutes.

16) **Reach for Toes in the Sky:**

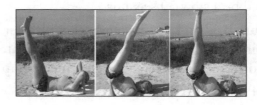

Lay on your back and hold your legs straight up while you reach to touch your toes with stiff arms. (Work to consciously elevate your heart rate. Keep your ab muscles tight the entire three minutes while you do 100 repetitions.)

17) **Scissor Kicks:**

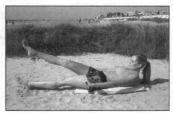

Lay on your back and keep your legs elevated and stiff while you alternately raise the left leg and lower the right leg.

18) **Shake the OJ:** Swing one gallon orange juice bottle from over your head to your knees 100 times.

19) **Side Scissors:**

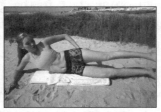

Lay on your side and raise your top leg as high as you can while keeping your leg stiff.

20) **Side Torso Lift:**

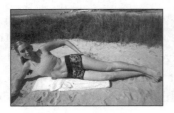 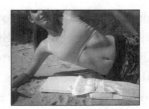

In the first picture see CJ's hip touching the ground but in the second picture she has elevated her torso.

21) **Side Plank Hip Elevation**: Similar to the Side Torso Lift, lay on your right side with your right elbow bent to be directly under your shoulder. Now instead of focusing on your torso, raise your hips to heaven. Keep your knees bent and your legs touching. Tighten your abdominal muscles each time your raise your hips, and keep your head in alignment with your spine.

22) **Squat Pops**: Hold onto a rail and slowly squat as low as you can, then quickly pop back up with enough force that your feet barely leave the ground.

23) **Stair Climber**: Run up four flights of stairs (100 steps) at the office.

24) **Supermans**: The endurance exercise that you perform by laying down prone (face to the ground) and lifting up your heels together and your arms in front of you for three minutes, or work up to that duration.

25) **Trot** around your house four times in three minutes.

The key component in the Energy Surge is to raise your heart rate while also activating as many muscles as possible. As Nike says, "Just do it!"

Aerobic Exercise

Aerobic exercise is the only exercise that consumes fat as the primary fuel. The US Surgeon General advises that this must be done for 30 minutes every other day. It should be easy and enjoyable. Things that might inhibit this exercise could include exercising at too high of intensity, not having social interaction (if needed), or perhaps a negative exercise experience in the past. Over 22% of the world population are overweight including 67% percent of the adult population in the US. These people have not been successful in obtaining permanent weight loss because they did not have the unique formula for their unique needs. Now you have that formula!

Exercise is different than mere activity when it either raises the heart rate for a prolonged period of time (i.e. bicycling for 20 minutes at 75% of maximum heart rate vs. walking through the shopping mall at a lower heart rate). Such cycling is low intensity, aerobic conditioning that burns fat as the primary fuel. Exercise can also include targeted resistance training where instead of burning fat as fuel, it leaves the basal (baseline) metabolic rate higher for a few hours. This can be accomplished by lifting a 2 lb. dumbbell for 20 repetitions (which also helps in making the muscle tissue denser) or you can lift a 10 lb. dumbbell four times. These two examples show movement of the same amount of weight but have drastically different outcomes. Which is easier?

To start your first day of easy exercise, first measure your **resting heart rate**. Sit quietly in a chair for five minutes and then count how many times your heart beats in 15 seconds and multiply by 4. Write down your resting heart rate. Then calculate your **aerobic target heart rate** by completing the following calculation: 220 − Age = B. Then B x .75 = aerobic target heart rate. Let's say you're 40 years old. Then: 220 − 40 = 180. 180 x .75 = 135 beats per minute. This is your target rate. In this phase it is always better to be lower than this number rather than having a higher heart rate.

Training with a heart rate higher than the aerobic threshold works the cardiovascular system and consumes glucose as the primary fuel. Both exercises are beneficial if your primary care physician approves it, but they have different goals and outcomes, and cardiac training is more difficult than fat loss training. Which do you want and what is your primary goal?

Resistance Training

In continuing our first day of easy exercise, you need to decide if you want resistance training or aerobic training. If you choose an **Easy Resistance Routine**, then you can use the following example of an easy full body resistance regime. This should be done continuously and only stopped to change positions or quickly drink a cup of water that you have beside your workout area. Start by drinking 8 oz. water and then proceed with the following exercises.

LEGS/TORSO

1) **Squats** Hold a 2 lb. dumbbell (DB) in each hand. With your back to a smooth wall, squat down and back up 20 times. In doing this maneuver, make sure to inhale on the way down and exhale on the way back up. (An easy way to remember which is which is that you will blow yourself up.) You should try to squat to a depth where your knees are bent in a 45 degree angle. Keep your head up by "pointing your nose above the horizon," not the ceiling and not the floor. Do 20 repetitions for a good start.

2) **Hip Lifts**

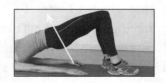

You will do the next set of exercises on your exercise pad or bed (remove all sheets and blankets that might get in your way if you are on your bed). Lay supine (tummy up) on the floor and place one of your 2 lb. DB on your tummy. Then feel the back of your legs as you push your heels down and raise your hips ½ inch. (This exercise is actually better on the floor if you are comfortable there.) Exhale all of the air out of your lungs as you lift your hips. The glutes (butt) and back muscles will be activated too, but the hamstrings will be the primary (agonistic), action muscle. Do this 20 times.

3) Ab Hold

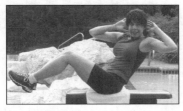

Sit on a bench or exercise mat. Lift your feet off the ground while touching your knees. Now hold this position as you move your hands back behind your head and hold this pose like Adele does so well!

4) Calf Raises

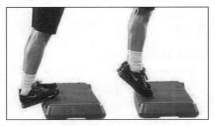

The calf muscle (gastrocnemius) has medial and lateral heads. To activate this muscle safely, get a 2 x 4 board and place it on the ground, preferably in front of a stair step with a handrail. Now place the DB in your right hand and place your right foot on the board with the ball of your foot (2nd metatarsals) right on the edge of the board. (See picture.) Lower your heel and inhale, then raise your heel as high as you can while exhaling all the air out of your lungs. Do this 20 times for each leg.

5) Isometric Gracilis, Groin Crunch

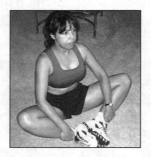

Isometric means muscles contract but the body does not move. While seated on the floor, place one DB between the heels of your shoes. Lock your feet into this parallel position and squeeze the DB between your feet. This is an isometric exercise because while you are activating the groin muscles (gracilis), there is no body movement. Do this 20 times.

CHEST/ARMS

1) Incline Chest Press

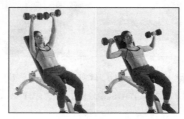

Sit, leaning back slightly in a wooden chair, and with a 2 lb. DB in each hand, bring your hands up to above your chest with the tips of the DB facing each other. (See picture.) Raise the DB in that fixed position for 20 repetitions. On every movement of the weight upward, you should exhale (blow up to the weight). Then on the way down (slowly) inhale a full volume of air. After 20 reps, stop and change the DB alignment to the hammer grip. Now complete another 20 reps and remember to keep exhaling as you push the weight to the sky.

2) **Back Row**

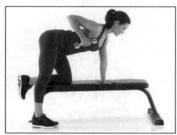

For a simple back exercise, kneel one leg onto a chair and with one hand let the DB go almost all of the way to the ground. Then lift the weight up as far as you can. Again exhale as you lift the weight each of the 20 reps. This exercise will activate many back, shoulder, and triceps muscles.

3) **Shoulders Extension**

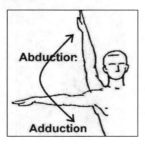

To activate these shoulder muscles, you will be standing and lifting the DB in abduction (moving away from body), which equals both arms away. First, stand with DB in the hammer position by your side and lift the DB to your eye level. (Exhale on the way up.) Complete 20 repetitions and then drink a cup of water. Holding the DB in hammer position again, elevate your hands from your side to shoulder level. As always it is important to exhale on the "action arm" of this movement, which is when you are lifting the dumbbell.

4) **Biceps Curls**

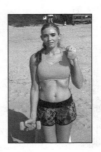

Stand and hold the DB in the supine position (as if you are holding a soup bowl) and fully curl your fist towards your chin while you keep your elbows locked against your side. Do this flat curl 20 times; and if you have lots of energy, complete another 20 repetitions with the DB in the hammer position.

5) **Triceps Extension**

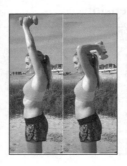

Remain standing and without resting lift the dumbbells above your head with a hammer grip position. Your knuckles should be touching and then let the weight drop behind your head. Now lift up and exhale forcefully as you complete your first of 20 repetitions.

Congratulations! You have just lifted over 800 lbs. of total weight in your continuous 20-minute "mega-set" exercise routine! Now drink another glass of water as you stretch any muscle that is fatigued or tired. (See chapter 12 on stretching.)

When you get comfortable in this routine after a month, then you can increase the challenge by increasing the repetitions by five per exercise. Then after using that regime for a month, the next change can be accomplished by changing to a larger weight (i.e. from 2 lbs. to 3 lbs.), and use this weight with the original 20 repetitions.

DIGEST THIS

This chapter shows all of the exercises you would ever need to gain the ideal physique and keep that stature forever! Just do any one of these exercises vigorously for 2-3 minutes a few times a day. If you want variation then choose a different exercise for the next month.

7

Natural Foods for Higher Energy

"One month after I finished a crash diet (the last of many), I was heavier than when I started! After the first 90 days with Doc, I had lost 20% of my initial Body Summation score and instead of rebounding, I continued to lose fat. After five years I am permanently 25% less than my initial Body Sum Score!'"
(Estella R., Corpus Christi, Texas)

Natural foods are the "N" in PEN. The fuel we take into our bodies determines how and what will be consumed as 1) energy, 2) used for building new cellular structures, or 3) is stored as fat. Natural nutrition is consuming products that have not been processed or modified. Ask "Did God put this on the planet." (And we won't get into genetically modified foods!)

Organic food is the ideal ingredient in this component for downsizing, but cost and availability often impair our choice of organic foods. However, eating fresh, unprocessed foods will be equally beneficial for your initial RightSize program. It is easy to think of eating raw fruits and vegetables or cooking foods without processed ingredients, but it is important to understand the functions of the nutrients in food and the metabolism of fats and sugars. This chapter will also give recommendations for planning the right fuel types (think of it as octane) and the right volume (how often should you fill up). What are your molecular needs?

Nutrients

The following are six essential nutrients that our bodies need to operate:

- **Carbohydrates** are used as immediate fuel.
- **Fats** are needed for cell covers (epithelium) and organ insulation. This can be fuel.
- **Proteins** provide the structural framework that our bodies need continually.
- **Fiber** assists in the digestion process.
- **Vitamins** are involved in chemical regulation like vitamin D to increase calcium absorption.
- **Water** is needed for most body functions as well as transporting nutrients throughout the body.

The Food and Drug administration has a useful website www.ChooseMyPlate.gov. for balancing one's intake of these dietary aspects. The following are their descriptions:

DIETARY CARBOHYDRATES are substances containing carbon, hydrogen, and oxygen. These substances can be broken down into sugars. The function of the carbohydrates is to provide energy for cellular work, maintain cell structure, generate heat, regulate fat, and assist in protein metabolism. The type of carbohydrate is determined by the heat generated through metabolism of these nutrients. A calorie is the heat required (or generated) to increase one gram of water by one degree Celsius. The calories needed for optimal functioning are estimated to be 2,000/day, depending on body size and activity level.

The average American consumes an estimate 3,900 calories/day, almost twice the needed calories per day with variation for gender and level of daily activity. If we are eating the wrong processed foods and more than we can digest, then it will be stored as fat. It has been shown that every two decades the average consumption increases by 700 calories. This means that in the next twenty years, our population of obese and overweight people will rise.

Simple carbohydrates (carbs) are the mono-saccharides and di-saccharides formed by simple sugar molecules and have little nutritive value. Such carbs are glucose, fructose, galactose, or combinations of those sugars. An apple is a simple carbohydrate. **Complex carbohydrates** are the valuable fuels, which are three or more sugar molecules linked together such as starches, dextrins, and glycogen. Complex carbs such as grains or seeds also include dietary fibers, which are actually not digested but used to process digestion of other food stuffs. These are plant products.

The next variable in carbohydrates is whether they are soluble or not. **Solubility** is the property that allows a particle to be dissolved into a liquid or gas. Sugar is soluble because it can fully dissolve into water, but fiber is not. Variables that affect a component's solubility are heat (temperature), volume, pressure, molecular polarity (how fast can the molecules be removed to mix). The rate or speed of solution is important. So if a substance is easily soluble, then it will require low energy for breakdown and will therefore be consumed easily without requiring high energy or work for breakdown, like sugar in water. But substances that are insoluble require greater energy for breakdown; or like fiber or fat, they will not be broken down.

DIETARY FATS OR LIPIDS are necessary and have multiple complex roles in a body's function. First, fats are required for the cell linings so they are necessary for cell structure and integrity. Fats are also needed to protect the organs and can be thought of as shock absorbers. However, excessive ingestion of fats can lead to a "fatty heart," in which case it will keep a body from its optimal function. The heart muscles are made to contract and pump blood; but since fats cannot contract, they impair the muscular contraction. Fats are also needed for roles as carriers of vitamins A, D, E, and K.

Fats can be used for fuel but in order for that to happen, aerobic exercise is required because the maximum oxygen intake is required to break down fats. This will be explained in greater detail in Chapter 13, but think of long endurance athletes who train for marathons, century bicycle rides (100 miles), or endurance swimming. These athletes have low body fat because of their continual, prolonged, low intensity aerobic exercise, which consumes fat as the primary fuel. Saturated fatty acids are long molecular chains that are difficult to cleave and break down. That is why saturated fatty acids are carried as molecules through the blood and can clog arteries (atherosclerosis).

DIETARY PROTEINS are complex organic compounds with the same elements as in sugars, but proteins also contain nitrogen and amino acids. Sugars are often circular structures and fat molecules have long single-chain structures (see figure 3), but the molecular structure of protein is often a "ball" of amino acid chains which have the greatest structure. (See Figure 3 below.)

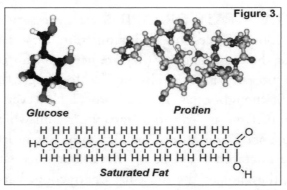

The function of protein includes building structures of bones, muscles, internal organs, hair, nails, and skin. Proteins also repair such structures and form active molecules such as enzymes for initiating reactions, hormones, and antibodies. These structures are also important for the normal balance of body fluids. These can be broken down as an energy source. A healthy diet with sufficient protein is important so that the body is not breaking down muscle as fuel while fats are being stored. The old adage "muscle turns into fat" is totally incorrect, but muscle atrophy (decrease in size and strength) often occurs simultaneously with fat expansion.

The types of proteins are differentiated by the type and number of amino acids. The 20 amino acids are building blocks. Nine essential amino acids are essential because your body cannot produce them. The body does not store amino acids so these essential amino acids must be ingested every day. One then may question, which protein is the most complete? The answer is the egg. The egg contains all 20 amino acids. While the egg contains all amino acids, it is interesting that only about 10% of a full egg is actually protein.

VITAMINS facilitate chemical reactions; however, vitamins provide no energy. Vitamins exist in both water and fat soluble types. The purpose of vitamins is to promote growth and stability in various life stages ranging from pregnancy to reducing osteoporosis in the elderly stage. Some vitamins also serve as antioxidants, which help reduce the cascade of erroneous cell replication that could become cancerous.

The primary vitamins, and their functions and food sources are listed in the table below.

VITAMIN	FUNCTION	FOOD SOURCES
Vitamin A	Renews eyes and skin	Liver, milk, cheese
Vitamin B1	Energy absorption	Whole grains
Vitamin B2	Energy production	Poultry, beef, liver, eggs
Vitamin B3	Use fat for energy	Mushrooms, peanut butter, fish, poultry
Vitamin B6	Produce glycogen	Potato, bananas
Vitamin B12	DNA structure	Milk, cheese, rice or soy
Biotin	Convert protein to carbs	Sweet potatoes
Vitamin C	Prevent cell damage	Citrus fruits, cantaloupe, cabbage, cauliflower, broccoli
Vitamin D	Transport calcium	Dairy products, eggs, fish
Vitamin E	Cell structure atherosclerosis	Yellow and green vegetables, Oatmeal, wheat germ, almonds, vegetable oils
	immune system	Avocados, leafy green vegetables, almonds
Folate	DNA structure	Asparagus, beets, broccoli,

		brussel sprouts, corn, peas, orange juice
Iron	Oxygen transport	Peas, egg yolk, fish
Vitamin K	Creates proteins to clot bleeding	Broccoli, collards, kale, soybeans, spinach, turnips,

MINERALS are indestructible inorganic structures listed on the chemical periodic table. The macro minerals include calcium, chloride, magnesium, phosphorus, potassium, sulfur, and sodium. Again water is the most important nutrient, particularly for all chemical reactions in your body, including breaking down fats. Examples of minerals in our diet are calcium from milk and copper from seafood or nuts.

The true bottom line of why optimal, natural nutrition is important can be understood with the fuel and fire analogy of one's metabolism. When a small flame is doused with a quickly consumable fuel (like gasoline), the flame bursts high but quickly reduces back. When swallowing a tablespoon of sugar, it will not have a lasting effect on raising the basal metabolic rate. However, placing a slow burning fuel on the fire will help increase the flame and continue it at an elevated rate. Eating whole, unprocessed food full of the optimal nutrients will help keep an elevated basal metabolic rate.

ANTIOXIDANTS are important for preventing disease and the following are the top foods containing antioxidants, proven in medical research:

- Blackberries
- Walnuts
- Strawberries
- Artichoke hearts
- Cranberries
- Raspberries
- Pecans

- Blueberries
- Ground clover
- Dark grapes
- Dark veggies
- Sweet potatoes
- Green tea (see more in Chapters 7 and 8)
- Whole grains

For optimal nutrition and balance, one can use the current FDA site, www.ChooseMyPlate.gov. This is a tremendous resource and has information on dishes, tracking, calorie calculations, eating tips (from vegetarians to eating out), and much more. This website was used successfully by subjects in a study led by Dr. Willis and Dr. Smith in 2012. The old Food Pyramid, www.FoodPyramid.com, also has volumes of delicious, healthy recipes. Recipes and tips on slow cooked meals can be found in Chapter 17.

How Much Should You Eat?

This category of using Natural foods allows one to eat as much as they want of natural, organic, and unprocessed foods. The benefit of natural foods is that they trigger the metabolic feedback of feeling satiated. This means your body will tell you when you are full compared to several noted weight loss foods or low calorie ingredients that do not give your body such feedback.

In the portion-size category, one must eat only 1.5 total cups per each of six meals, but in the Natural category you can feel comfortable eating up to one cup of vegetables, plus one cup of fruits, one cup of milk, and 4-6 oz. of protein such as grilled chicken. (Remember not to use any processed toppings in the grilling, so baste with lime and organic, natural honey or homemade salsa.) Eating all Natural food products can allow 2-3 times the volume of food to be ingested as allowed in the Portion-size category. Se when you need more food (fuel), then eat Natural to RightSize!

Accelerate Fat Loss

The following are foods shown to accelerate fat loss:

- **Asparagus** (folic acid and glutathione)
- **Apricots** (Vitamins A and C, fiber, iron, calcium)
- **Apples** (Increased peristalsis, detoxification,
    and better digestion)
- **Beets** (binds to fats, decreases water retention, and reduces colon cancer)
- **Carrots** (beta-carotene and binds to cholesterol)
- **Chili Pepper** (increases metabolism—burn, baby, burn!)
- **Cucumber** (natural diuretic and increases metabolism
- **Garlic** (diuretic and increases metabolism with
    antibiotic effects)
- **Grapefruit** (increases metabolism and proven
    to help fat loss)
- **Green Tea** (increases oxidation for increased fat breakdown)
- **Onion** (binds to food for faster breakdown)

DIGEST THIS

Use the Natural food products as the best fuel to give you the energy for a continuous fire. Instead of throwing gas on the fire and creating an explosion, simply forecast your food and plan to eat quality products every two hours like planning when you have to fuel up for a long drive.

8

Eat Often for Better Digestion

"I first had to realize that there is nothing wrong with being BBW (a big, beautiful woman), but there was a problem that multiple rolls of fat are not healthy. Doc said to 'think about the inside' and my metabolic fire, and he would be the only person to know my external numbers (Body Summation Score). After five years, my Body Summation Score is literally half of what it was when I started MY formula to MY Success! Doc is my angel!" *(Rachel P., Midland, Texas)*

Research has shown that eating portion sizes (of the same total volume of food) yields greater fat loss. This was proven in a matched study of athletes who were performing the same daily exercises, and ate the same exact daily food products and the same total volume of food. It showed that if you eat 36 oz. of food over three meals versus eating 36 oz. of food over six meals, the latter yields a higher metabolic rate. Eating more frequent, smaller portions helps our bodies digests the food more completely and stores less fat! (All clinical, research studies are listed in the Bibliography at the end of this text. # 31-36 in Bibliography)

The FDA and Center for Disease Control (CDC)

teamed up to sponsor a broad investigation of "Portion Sizes: Now and Then." (#43 in Bibliography) The bottom line is that the Western world's average portion size has increased substantially in the past two decades. One book and several studies may give the right template for such balance.

In *The Metabolism Advantage,* (2006) Dr. Berardi recommends eating every two to three hours. His book says,

> Each time you eat, you stimulate your metabolism for a short period of time, which means that the more often you eat, the more you'll increase your metabolism. Eating every 2 to 3 hours feeds muscle and starves fat. By eating frequently, you reassure your body that you aren't going to starve; that food will always be available. Skipping breakfast, eating only a sandwich for lunch, and pigging out at dinner, on the other hand, frightens your body into storing fat, just in case your next meal never comes.

Dr. Dan Benardot's research at Georgia State University clearly showed that the more frequent eating patterns yielded lower body fat and higher muscle mass. In a study he said that eating small, frequent meals and consuming fluid at regular intervals are optimal and that "There is good evidence that weight rebound is a common aspect of dieting, affecting up to 80% of dieters." Dr. Benardot's research has shown energy deficits from peak and valley meal plans (i.e. eating three times a day with 5 hours between meals). Such diets showed the highest body fat percentages.

Portion Size as Fuel

Think of the portion-size component as a wood-burning

fire. Picture yourself alone in the cold mountains and you only have a cubic meter stack of wood and kindling to burn for 24 hours. Will you burn it all at once? Of course you would not, but you will slowly feed the fire with small additions of wood throughout the day. If you put too much on the fire at any time, it will also generate greater quantities of ash, which would not be completely consumed by the fire. So feeding the fire of your metabolism keeps the fire burning and does not leave excess ash (fat) behind.

Pyramid Meals increase the quantity of foods we eat until our third or fourth is the largest before we continually reduce the volume of food we are eating. That is a sequence of meals every 2-3 hours, which equals five meals in the normal day. The pyramid aspect can be linked again to the flame and fuel analogy. When one first starts the flame, we do not need to saturate the flame with fuel. (An Energy Surge before the meal will speed up your metabolism even more.)

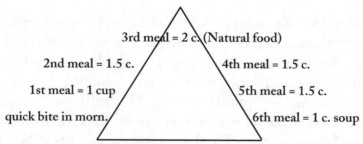

A common practice in bodybuilding is to start with the smallest, lightest meal and progress until the third meal, the largest and packed with natural nutrients. Meal sizes then decrease until the last meal (6th), which is small and light (similar to the first meal).

Interesting studies have looked at changes in portion size

and lack of awareness by the subjects or consumers. In a laboratory (Dilberti 2001), subjects were fed a 50% greater serving of a pasta dish; and in a post meal survey, only 7% of the subjects noted the increased portion size! Portion size has been proclaimed as an integral factor in weight loss, but consumers may not be conscious of the appropriate volumes of food. While some restaurants admit that they consciously feed patrons more than appropriate volumes of food, 69% of customers report that they regularly eat all the food served. That is interesting because 67% of the USA are overweight. Does being taught to clean our plates affect our pattern of eating as adults?

Again research has shown that while one should eat a larger total volume of food but in smaller, more numerous doses. Dr. Rolls systematic review study cited that when large portions are available, people continue to eat more. Using the fuel analogy, people are taking on more fuel than they need; and if not used during activity, it will be stored as fat.

Consuming portion-sized meals was further proven by Dr. Foster and colleagues from Temple University in a study of 69 obese patients with Type II Diabetes (Foster 2009). The subjects were categorized as obese because they had a BMI ≥ 39. The subjects' mean age was 52 years of age and half of them were African Americans. One group consumed only portion-sized meals, four times a day for three months, and the other group only received education with no control over the portion sizes of food.

After three months there was a significant difference in all variables including the following:

• Weight decreased for the portion-size group by 18 lbs. vs 0 lbs. for the education only group.

• Waist circumference was reduced 3.3 inches for the portion-size group vs. 0 in. for the education only group.
• Lowered blood pressure for the portion-size group
• Reduced HbA1c (blood glucose over time) for the portion-size group
• Systolic blood pressure was reduced by the portion-size group
• Triglycerides and total cholesterol were reduced by the portion-size group

Then the education group was directed into eating portion-sized meals, and they also showed a sequential change in weight, waist circumference, etc. Eating portion-sized meals reduces weight and waistline, and improves one's health.

DIGEST THIS

Eat smaller portions. For example, one meal you can eat is one CLIFF protein bar. (A patient called these "Snickers on steroids!") Then for your next feeding try a Natural Nutrition meal that has no boundaries on the quantities that you can eat. Eat a kids' meal for the explosive metabolism of a young child. Having just a two-hour interval following a Portion size feeding will keep you from temptation while also keeping your metabolic fire high!

9

Let's Get Real

"At my 40th birthday I was outwardly proclaiming how wonderful I felt, but that was excluding my body which was overweight. I had successfully lost weight on the Atkins diet, the Raw Diet, Weight Watchers, and dozens more, but I could never translate those programs into retention until I met Doc who showed me the simple, baby steps to permanent weight loss of 40 lbs. and four dress sizes!" *(Rachelle W., Austin, Texas)*

Formula Layout

First, consult your primary care physician and ask for a complete blood count to measure your starting point. Next, complete the Body Summation evaluation and measurement. You can ask the staff at your Doctor's office (or a trusted, supportive relative or friend) to help you complete this form. That will give you a concrete, analytical starting point that is more accurate and inclusive than a bathroom scale (although weight is included in that score). It also gives better, descriptive feedback along your pathway to RightSizing!

The Body Summation is the total of most all circumferences of your body which gives one a measurable, quantifiable measurement that is far more accurate than just weighing on the scale. You can find this form online or at back of book.

Plan Your Success to RightSize!

Begin your plan by conceptualizing that you will consume food in five "dining events." Think of this as taking in fuel to reach your RightSize destination!

DAY ONE: Start your day with low intensity cardiovascular exercise in the morning for 10 minutes (Target heart rate = (220-Age) x .75 = HR

- Eat one meal that is portion size controlled (P)
- Do one pre-meal Energy Surge (E)
- Eat one meal that is natural nutrition (N)
- Eat two meals of anything without pre-exercise

DAY TWO: Using PEN—make P four of out of your five dining events

- Add 2 cups of water in the morning to each day's routine.
- Do stretching (shoulders, biceps, triceps, quads, hamstrings, inner calf, outer calf muscles) in the evening for one minute each.

DAY THREE: Do all five dining events in the PEN protocol

- Add 20 minutes of low intensity exercise in the morning or evening.

DAY FOUR: Includes all five PEN selections and

stretching (shoulders, biceps, triceps, quads, hamstrings, inner calf, outer calf muscles) for one minute each .

DAY FIVE: All five dining events in the PEN protocol
• add 2 cups water while you perform Resistance exercise (see chapter 6)

DAY SIX: All five dining events in the PEN protocol
• Plus 20 minutes of low intensity exercise in the morning or evening

DAY SEVEN: Group activity (i.e. quick walking with your family or quiet bicycle rides) and one delicious treat or dessert for one feeding as your portion size selection. If you go to a restaurant just say, "I will just have a piece of the Decadent Chocolate Cake for my entrée." That is ALL you will eat for this portion size. It is best to eat nutritious food, but this is an example that works for weight loss.

You have read the scientific success of subjects who used portion control, frequent exercise, or natural nutritional components for significant benefits in fat loss, reduction of diabetes, and reduction of clinical risk factors for heart disease, diabetes, etc. The testimonies were the high points from thousands of people who have used these components to achieve fat loss. Now it is time to construct *your* plan, for your enjoyable, permanent RightSize.

First, you should consult your primary care physician, at least to tell them of your plan. Having your annual physical including blood panels would be ideal to show later how your fat loss has changed or you have reduced other risk factors like hyperlipidemia (high LDL), etc.

Next, you will track and document everything for the first month with an accountability partner for weekly follow up. Through the internet, my Certified Personal Trainers and I would enjoy being your professional consultants. Having your spouse, friend, or family member would be ideal too. (Remember, this needs to be an optimistic, supportive person who will give you the clear accountability for success.)

In the following pages you will see the testing summation forms and then the daily and weekly tracking forms. Take the initial testing form to your physician and then make a follow up appointment with your doctor's nurse or assistant for the second and third month for follow-up testing. Reward yourself for this accomplishment!

Plan and schedule to only have one large, formal meal per week but four meals per day in your first month. The formal meal is defined as a social, recreational event that includes food that may be prepared by someone else. An example of such a meal could be, Sunday dinner with your mom and dad or a hamburger cookout with your children's soccer teams. Your typical meals will be four to five times each day where you will eat food with the stipulation that it will either be a) a portion controlled volume of 1.5 cups (a two-handed cereal bowl of food; b) a meal preceded by 2-3 minutes at your target heart rate; or c) natural nutritional ingredients equaling one plate of food. An example of this would be ½ cup steamed green beans, ½ chicken breast, ½ cup brown rice, and one piece of bread that you made from scratch, not a mix.

You can have more than one social meal each week, but the second such un-controlled meal MUST be immediately preceded with an exercise that raises your heart rate to your target zone for 2-3 minutes. If you have a business lunch, before the meeting, quickly go up and down the stairs for 2-3 minutes. When they ask about it, just say, "My doctor told me to do this." Later you can tell them how your RightSize formula gave you a new, lean, permanent physique with optimal blood pressure and blood glucose.

Regular Easy Exercise

Tracking your food intake and exercise is important to find the exact formula that best suits your schedule and gives you the most dramatic weight loss. After your first day, write down a pilot plan for your first week. Which days will be your cardio/aerobic training (where and when)? Then determine if you have special events that you will need to proceed with exercise. It is also important that you write down a score for your performance (i.e. 1-10) so that you can correlate what you felt was the most successful. Our model and victor CJ recommends completing one set of stretching poses and then to walk briskly (with elevated heart rate) for 20 minutes. This accomplishes multifaceted training of both resistance (muscle activation to reach and hold your positions), flexibility, and cardio vascular training.

Living in the new healthy environment will definitely benefit children too. Children are motivated and inspired by their parents. If you are living a healthy lifestyle, your children will follow. What is your motivation for starting this formula? What control mechanisms do you need to have so that you do not splurge and binge detrimentally? When you encounter a tempting situation, exercising portion control will help you. Instead of eating a 5-course meal, start with dessert. This may satiate your need to over-indulge. You will encounter a host of obstacles but just be determined to work through them all.

One reader asked if it were better to exercise for six minutes, five times a week, or one day for 30 minutes. I believe the answer resides in the optimal pattern of exercise that we need to follow. When I was a boy we ran, played, and unknowingly exercised all day long. Recess and PE were high points of our days in elementary school, and even on birthdays we'd have races and challenges. The frequency of exercise is more important than one single bout, and at the same time, don't forget that aerobic exercise is the only exercise that will preferentially consume fat as fuel. So my answer is "Yes, and..." Let's do both!

Goals are most effective if they are written, specific, measurable, acceptable, time-specific, and can have random period evaluations. Write down your overall goal (e.g., back to dress size 8) and plan on monthly, appropriate goals to reach in a reasonable period of time. How long did it take you to gain the weight? Then it will take roughly half that time to reach your new, lifetime goal with permanence!

Accelerate Your Success

When eating, remember TIPS: Tease Increases Powerful Stimulation for your metabolism. When you tease your body to want more but do not fulfill that desire, you increase metabolism. When teasing your body, always think of the total volume you are eating and the total volume in your stomach.

1. **Tease your body** (one bite and wait 10 minutes to eat)

2. **Increase your caloric value** (by not eating processed sugar based high fructose corn syrup (HCF), you will train

your body to use the quality fuel better than just saving the cheap fuel as fat! Think of how easy it is for the body to turn a slice of a pound cake versus a strawberry. Both are sweet and delicious but the pound cake that is primarily flour and sugar is easily converted into glucose and unless used is converted into fat. Where a strawberry actually requires more calories of energy to break it down than it delivers as fuel, so the net glucose going to fat deposition is zero.

3. **Powerful stimulation** comes in many ways:
   • Prevent your stomach from ever being empty. (When you stomach is empty, the body goes on survival mode and lowers the metabolic rate to the lowest possible levels!)
   • Push Back! (Enjoy leaving food on your plate or share one entree with your sweetie. Then snack on the leftovers later!)

4. **Stimulate your appetite**
Take Tease tastes at the grocery store when they offer samples. When you see the Girl Scout cookie stands, buy a pack, take one out, and immediately give the pack back to the kids to eat! One cookie will raise your metabolism, whereas eating the whole pack will slow your total time of digestion, cause discomfort, and slow down your success.

5. **Eat with a slow rhythm and small bites,**
Let the flavors slowly dissolve in your mouth. When listening to music, which genre do you prefer? Think of your food as an instrument that builds and crescendos. Will you be playing a long musical and need low level energy or a bright aria that will delight many senses?

Think about the strength, power, and stamina that both a horse evokes and its rider shares. Will eating a fluffy tart or grabbing a bright, dense, red apple empower such a ride? I know what Secretariat would choose! What fuel reminds you of the greatest pleasure? (Not Christmas dinner that leaves one stuffed.) Use this TIPS concept in your food choices as well!

DIGEST THIS

You can eat anything if you make the plan of how and when you will eat more fuel for a better burn!

10

Tease, not Overload

"We had a combined weight of 660 lbs., which equaled twice our college weights. We thought Doc's program was too easy to last, but it has taken us through several Christmas food orgies and kept us at a total of 300 lbs!" *(Rebecca is now 120 lbs. and Mike is 180 lbs. from Abilene, Texas)*

Teasing your body into gaining a faster metabolic rate and here are simple, proven tips to raise your metabolism.

Move First thing in the morning. It has been shown in abundant studies that performing a quick exercise routine when you first wake up accelerates the metabolism for a few hours. While it is still elevated, do other things to keep the metabolic rate as high as possible.

One Bite ASAP—eating one bite of fruit or meat will significantly elevate the metabolism. When we sleep, the body is fasting and has the lowest metabolic level. Eating just one bite is a tease that turns up the fire on your metabolism. Eat one bite ASAP or immediately after your exercise and then leisurely get ready for work before having a slow breakfast.

Eat Breakfast because not eating breakfast throws your body into a survival mode where the metabolic rate and energy are significantly reduced. Tell your body that it will have ample food throughout the day so that it keeps the fires burning as high as possible!

Turn Up the Heat on your food. Capsaicin is the chemical compound that makes chili peppers hot. Eating a tablespoon of chopped red or green chili peppers achieves a temporary spike in the metabolism up to 23%. Drs. Shin and Moritani (2007) found in their study that consuming capsaicin, green tea, and chicken essence tablets raised the thermogenic effect by triggering a metabolic "fight or flight" sympathetic response. This raised the basal metabolic rate without increasing heart rate or blood pressure. Eat some chili peppers on your burger or add red peppers on pizza for a bit of metabolic heat.

Women, Pump Some Iron because iron deficiency causes the metabolism to plummet. If you have low iron, then your body will carry less oxygen to the muscles. Less efficient muscle activity will lower your basal metabolic rate as a protection mechanism. So eat more beans, dark leafy greens like spinach and bok choy, and broccoli.

Go Fish or at least consume more fish oil vitamins to increase your metabolism. Several studies have shown that consuming six grams of fish oil vitamins can increase weight loss and accelerate weight loss with exercise.

Eat More Energy Foods such as whole grains, beans, vegetables, and fruits. The higher quality fuel you consume, the stronger and higher the metabolic flame.

Water for Weight Loss was evaluated in a clinical study, and it showed that subjects who drank 8 glasses a day vs 4 glasses per day lost more weight. However, too much water can also be a problem that causes hyponatremia (low sodium in the blood), which contributes to congestive heart failure, kidney and liver failures and pneumonia.

Snack Attacks are good if they are signals from your body to eat more good stuff! Throw out the chips and Snickers and pick up an apple or banana every two hours. This will keep you from being hungry and will keep the metabolic fire high.

Protein for Lunch is good and a pyramid strategy of eating the most nutrient dense proteins in the middle of your day has been used for many years. If you are not focused on portion size or exercise, then you could eat sequentially increasing and decreasing food volumes like 4 oz., 8 oz., 12 oz., 8 oz., and 4 oz. throughout the day.

Sip Coffee and Drink Water Drinking an 8 oz. glass of water after every cup of coffee has a thermogenic effect. Coffee can be a diuretic, but following it with a cool glass of water will help negate the detrimental effects of coffee by itself.

Fresh Brewed Green Tea can be consumed for increased metabolism. While most studies link the increased metabolism effects of tea to caffeine, Dr. Duloo led a study which found that "green tea extract stimulates brown adipose tissue thermogenesis." In an energy expenditure study comparing green tea vs. caffeine vs. placebo, they found that there was a significant difference with the green tea. Duloo (2000) and colleagues concluded that green tea has thermogenic properties more powerful in fat breakdown than just the caffeine in the tea.

Taurine (energy drinks) can speed up your metabolism and may help burn fat. Studies have also shown that taurine helps reduce inflammatory reactions and works effectively as an antioxidant. The studies exploring increased fat breakdown with taurine are promising.

Reducing Stress can increase your metabolism significantly. Exercise and weight loss have been shown beneficial in reducing stress so you are on the right pathway. Other things that can help one reduce stress are the following:

- **Take time to breathe:** Schedule a few times each day to get away from noise, and deeply and slowly breathe in as much air as possible and then gently exhale the air in a tiny wind stream.

- **Be present:** Shake off the past and don't worry about the future. You are here, alive, and remarkable TODAY!

- **Volunteer:** Giving of your time to others whether it is at church or a Big-Brother, Big-Sister program will refill you and give you joy that supersedes stress.

- **Pray or meditate:** This gives a centering, grounding effect and often lets me be quiet so that I can hear the answers to my questions. Use this time to remember your positive attributes.

- **Relax physically:** You can do numerous things to help your body relax such as wrapping a warm towel around your neck or getting a massage. Have your special someone rub your hands and feet with a warming balm.

• **Get moving:** Doing an Energy Surge does not have to be just before a few meals. If your business day is stressed then just take a 2 minute break to run some stairs or do 100 jumping jacks! Exercise has been proven effective in reducing stress.

• **Laugh it up!** My friend and mentor Dr. Patch Adams uses laughter as the best medicine! Laughter releases endorphins, which reduce stress hormones. Learn a joke or wear a squeaky red nose for no reason! If you just walk through a grocery store with a big red nose on, you will bring lots of quiet giggles and laughs!

• **Sleep more!** The appetite center is in the hypothalamus of the brain, and sleep directly influences the efficacy of this organ. Leptin is the appetite suppressant hormone in the hypothalamus, and Spiegel and colleagues (et al) showed that sleep deprivation decreases Leptin levels, thereby raising one's appetite.

DIGEST THIS

Teasing your body into gaining a faster metabolic rate is easy when you eat only one bite of chocolate and wait a few minutes before eating your meal. Unique foods and teas help accelerate your change with the easy RightSize program.

11

Activate the Change

"I had 'Hang-over' (which means my belly hung over my belt), but now I have a hard, flat stomach at 45 years of age!" *(James A., San Marcos, Texas)*

Dietary Supplements

Which vitamins have been proven to help in weight loss? Vitamin supplements brag about enormous, remarkable results, but with 100s of products on the market, which work? A study by Bell et al (2009) says there have only been 14 published clinical studies on vitamins and in those 14 studies, only three single ingredients were proven to be effective: chromium picolinate, green tea extract, and ma huang (ephedra). Here are descriptions of those supplements and others proven empirically to benefit weight loss through either raising the metabolism or enhancing the digestive system.

Chromium Picolinate has been shown to improve mood, appetite, carbohydrate metabolism, and glucose regulation, fasting blood glucose tests. (#40 in Bibliography). Limited evidence has shown **green tea** can be beneficial in reducing and preventing cardiovascular heart disease and reducing weight. **Ma huang** has since been banned by the FDA for safety in the United States because it has been shown to cause serious, even fatal, side effects such as heart attack, stroke, irregular heartbeats, and sudden death. The FDA has recommended that consumers not take ma huang.

A review by Bell, et al. showed that **Phaseolus vulgaris** and **hydroxycitric acid** can also have statistically significant effects in weight loss. The true bottom line is that dietary supplements may be beneficial in early stages, but they would not be effective for continual, long term change. The following are other supplements that can be used:

L CARNITINE is created in the liver and kidneys, and it is found in animal products, particularly red meat. It is a popular vitamin supplement for athletes and people who suffer from chronic slow metabolism. Carnitine's function is to carry fatty acids to the mitochondria, the powerhouse of muscle cells. For most people, the supplement L Carnitine helps raise the metabolism by giving more energy to the skeletal muscle fibers.

Carnitine deficiency is a genetic, metabolic disease that is treated with L Carnitine. See your physician if you are experiencing the following chronic, simultaneous symptoms: weakness in the hips, shoulders, upper arms, and legs combined with weak neck and jaw muscles, and a weak heart. In advanced cases, additional symptoms can include vomiting, growth retardation in children, and liver enlargement. If all of these symptoms are occurring together, go see your physician for easy testing that can determine if this is a metabolic disease or not.

CUMIN CYMINUM comes from an herb that is similar to parsley. It is often used in food from South America and Middle Eastern countries and has a unique aromatic fragrance. In a randomized, double-blinded, placebo trial (the highest level of experimental designs) by Taghizadeh, Memarzadeh, Asem, Esmaillzadeh (2015), they found subjects had significant weight loss after eight weeks, and there was a statistical difference from the subjects who consumed only the placebo tablets.

SEEDS In addition to natural foods and dietary supplements, seeds have empowered people trying to lose weight. Pomegranate seeds have vitamin C, are low in calories and high in fiber. Hemp seeds are rich in fiber and, through colonic stimulation and irritation, this substance accelerates food passage through the lower GI. Pumpkin seeds are rich in iron and protein and include the essential amino acids tryptophan and glutamate. Pumpkin seeds, while high in calories, have also been found to be antioxidants. Chia seeds are rich in Omega-3 and Omega-6 oils (which help carry out the Low Density Lipoproteins or LDL, bad fats). While these seeds have reported to increase energy levels for weight loss, there have been reported side effects of anxiety and an increased association with prostate cancer.

Wheat Germ is a good source of fiber and vitamin E. Flax seeds are dietary fibers, rich in micronutrients. These seeds have been shown beneficial in reducing cholesterol, but there were mixed results between men vs. women. Sesame seeds have been shown effective in reducing LDLs but sesame seed oils have also been shown to cause high incidences of allergic reactions in children.

HCG, HUMAN CHORIONIC GONADOTROPIN is a hormone produced in pregnancy to ensure that blood and nutrients reach the fetus. However, it is now being used for weight loss. This hormone has shown to substantially reduce the appetite. This is a pharmaceutical medication, available only through prescription.

While HCG can be beneficial for weight loss, it is important to realize that there are abundant, dangerous, and life-threatening side effects with such a treatment. Thermogenic products like Lipo-6 have not been adequately tested. One theory behind their use is that these products accelerate fat consumption during aerobic exercise. However, significant adverse effects have been reported, including tachycardia (rapid, elevated heart rate), headaches, and insomnia.

TEA

While caffeine has a pronounced effect on raising one's metabolism, there are both better drinks and limitations with all weight loss beverages. Here is a synopsis of the tea and coffee products that claim weight loss.

GREEN TEA EXTRACT is effective in weight loss and is also as an antioxidant, anticarcinogen, anti-inflammatory treatment. It helps remove lipids and lipid free radicals that cause excessive cell growth (cancer). The anti-inflammatory properties help enhance the digestive system, which again will consume more energy from the food digested rather than saving the energy as fat. Green tea was the subject of a randomized, double blind study. (A double blind study means neither the investigator nor the subjects know who is drinking the experimental vs. placebo products.)

Chen and colleagues (2015) examined high dose green tea extract compared to a control on 102 women with high BMI (>27) and a large waist circumferences (>31.5 in.). After 12 weeks the women who drank the high dose green tea extract had a significant change in BMI and waist circumference while the control subjects did not. The resounding finding was that cholesterol was reduced by more than 5% in the subjects who drank the high dose tea.

In a similar way, GINGER TEA has been shown to activate the digestive system while also reducing inflammation. A controlled trial was completed by Azimie et al (2014). They examined the effect three glasses of dark tea with cinnamon or ginger had versus control teas in patients with Diabetes Type II. While they did not use body composition testing as a variable, they found that it significantly lowered subjects LDL, HDL, and cholesterol compared to control subjects.

Coffee

While there has been repeated evidence that coffee can benefit weight loss, there is now new interest in Green Coffee's ability to reduce weight and fat volumes. Mullin (2015) wrote an interesting position paper on this product saying that caffeine may spark initial weight loss, but that increased caffeine consumption would not result in permanent weight loss.

Alcohol

The first rule in drinking alcohol with this program is to drink slowly. That means only one glass or wine, one beer, or one mixed beverage per hour. Also, alcohol is a diuretic. So for each serving of alcohol, you must drink a glass of water. Also our sleep quality when drinking is impacted. The answer for that is to stop all alcohol consumption three hours before bed.

Another thing to remember is that alcohol lowers one's testosterone so we need also perform the resistance training before a planned drinking event. When counting the value of energy derived from the drinks, red and white wine are the best. If you are planning on consuming more than one glass of wine a few times a week, then earlier in the day perform resistance training. For every glass of wine, also consume a full glass of water following the hour it takes you to consume the wine. Also eat before your drink.

DIGEST THIS

Supplements like L-carnitine and products like green tea will help elevate your metabolism for faster weight loss. These triggers won't solve the problem by themselves, but when combined with PEN, can accelerate your weight loss.

SECTION III

Your Best Body Forever

12

Muscle Stretching

"I had a chronic knee injury. Doc's program for knee rehabilitation has reduced my pain...and my waist by 12 inches...and kept it off!" *(Estella G., New Braunfels, Texas.* Taken from *Effective Orthopedic Rehab: Ten Steps to Complete Recovery* by Dr. Willis)

Stretching Techniques and Methods

Stretching is important when you are starting new exercise routines (even the Energy Surge) that can secrete lactic acid, which can give muscle soreness. Stretching also decreases the trend to overtrain. It increases blood flow to the muscles for recovery, and it increases muscle tone. Stretching also lets you cool down for a few minutes after exercising. The cool down plus stretching will reabsorb the lactic acid, which is generated through the muscular contractions, preventing muscle soreness the second day.

With this program you will be losing so much weight that you need to stretch to reconfigure your new body. The blanket rule for stretching is to hold each stretch repetition for 20–30 seconds where there is constant muscle tension. One should not try to pull too tightly because that can cause micro tears, and you should definitely avoid "bouncing" which can also cause significant tears of the muscle, connective tissues, and cross bridge muscle fibers of the muscle.

There are four main stretching techniques, and different techniques should follow different phases.

• **PRIMARY STRETCHING** uses the techniques of obtaining muscle tension and holding it for 20 to 30 seconds by using the opposing muscle (antagonist) or positioning to achieve the tension for stretching. This is the technique most often used by sports medicine in training athletes. One example would be a "groin stretch" where one sits with feet together, leaning forward, and uses the body position to make the groin (gracilius) muscle tense. (See the Prayer stretch.)

• **PASSIVE, STATIC STRETCHING** is a technique that uses gravity and/or position to gain the effect of gently stretching one's muscle fibers. This can best be described with the stretching of an elbow. The elbow is positioned, outstretched on a table (palm up) with one's wrist and forearm being pressed down only by gravity. Such a stretch is appropriate in the acute phase of treating injuries such as tennis elbow.

• **PRIMARY ASSISTED STRETCHING** uses the force of another person to achieve additional muscle tension. This technique should only be done with a trained physical therapist, athletic trainer, or a trained physician because it can easily result in compounding the injury being treated (Bibliography #1,2,8,15,16). An example of primary assisted stretching is for the hamstring, where one lays with his back on the ground (supine), and a partner raises one of the other person's legs for extra tension.

• PROPRIOCEPTIVE NEUROMUSCULAR FACILITATION (PNF) is the stretching used for increased force production in athletics. In this strength training technique, one stretches one muscle group intensely before performing a forceful contraction of that muscle group. This technique is only appropriate in the Recovery phase of rehabilitation or for advanced exercise training. An example of PNF is the Jump Squat used by high-jump athletes, right before their jump over the bar. In this example PNF is similar to Plyometric training that will be discussed later in this chapter.

Stretching, just like strength training, must advance gradually, and this can be done by using changes in the Frequency, Intensity, and Time of duration (FIT). This allows subtle variations for gradual progression, rather than just increasing the intensity of the stretch. FIT is another integral component of Stair Step progression, and utilization of this method will be described with clinical examples, starting in chapter 6, and it will also be discussed in chapter 13, regarding design of your rehabilitation program.

Stretches for Each Body Region
NECK/UPPER BACK

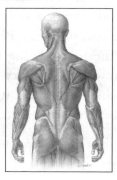

1) Self-Hug

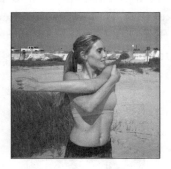

Sit or stand up straight and allow your shoulders and arms to relax. Extend both arms in front of you, and grab the left shoulder with your right hand. Cross your left arm beneath the right arm and grab your elbow. Pull the right elbow across your body, which makes your right hand move to the center of your back when in a full stretch. This is an effective trapezius stretch.

2) Sternocleidomastoid-Trapezius Stretch

This muscle group goes from behind your ear to your collar bone. Gently tilt your head to the side. After holding that position for 15 seconds, let your head roll forward to engage and stretch the trapezius (top shoulder to neck muscle).

3) Knee Tuck

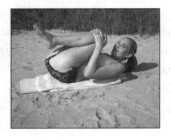

Simply lay on your back (supine) and pull your knees to your chest. Make sure to keep your head down on the stretching pad so that you do not strain your neck. As always, hold each stretch for 30 continual seconds.

4) Bend Over

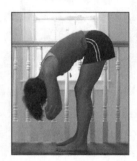

Grab both elbows and bend over to stretch your back muscles.

5) Back Bend

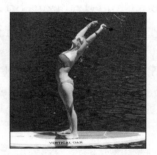

This will stretch the opposite (front) back and abdominal muscles, compared to the back bend exercise. Stand with feet one half meter apart, grab a bar or rail at 5 foot and push your abs forward while bending your shoulders back. Doing this on a balance board like Amy is doing is an amazing workout!

LOWER BACK
1) Hamstring Stretching

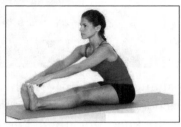

Begin by sitting on the mat with both legs extended, and extend your arms over the legs by bending farther at the waist. This will stretch the hamstrings and maintain each full tension stretch for 30 continuous seconds.

2) Back Extension Stretch

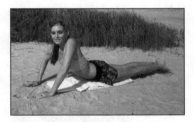

Lying face down (prone), crawl your hands to be beneath your shoulders and push up. Now let your hips descend to stretch.

3) Torque Knees to Chest Stretch

Start with the Knee Tuck position and extend one leg. Hold the leg out, pulling the tucked knee more closely before changing legs. Hold for 30 seconds.

4) Lumbar Rotation (Knee Flexed)

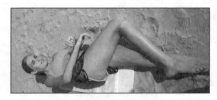

Begin laying supine on your pad with your feet on the pad and your knees bent to 90 degrees. Extend your arms laterally and bring your knees together. Then let both knees drape over to one side. Hold for 30 seconds and then return to the neutral, upright position for 30 seconds before draping over to the other side for 30 seconds.

SHOULDERS/PECS
1) Scapula Stretch

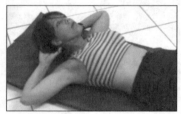

Lay on your back with your hands behind your head and elbows on the ground. Bring your fingers together behind your head. This will stretch your shoulder blade (scapula) muscles.

2) Lying Arm Abduction Stretch

While laying on your back (supine), reach your hands overhead at 2 o'clock and 10 o'clock with your elbows on the ground. Hold for 30 seconds and do two sets.

3) Pec Stretch (hands apart)

This is an easy wall stretch. Raise your upper arm (humerus) parallel to the ground and then flex your elbow to 90 degrees (make a right angle). Walk to a door and while holding that position, place the hand to elbow on the door jam and lean into the door to stretch the pectoral muscles.

UPPER ARM/ELBOW
1) Biceps Flexion Stretch with Rotation

Raise your elbow so that the humerus (upper arm bone) is parallel to the floor and aim your elbow in front of your body. Flex your biceps (curling motion) so that your fingertips can almost touch your shoulders and hold that for 30 seconds. After that initial stretch, repeat a second stretch with your thumb pointed to your shoulder for 30 seconds.

2) Triceps Extension Stretch

Place your elbow on a flat surface and extend your arm as far as you can (hold for 30 seconds). Then for the second 30-second stretch, sit in an office chair and drape your arm across the armrest with your elbow on the armrest pad. To activate this position, stretch your fingers in extension as if you were trying to touch the bottom of the chair with your fingertips.

3) **Prayer Stretch**

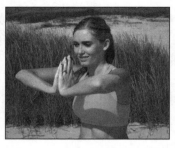

Bring your hands together in front of your chest, making the motion of a small child praying. To activate this stretch, raise your shoulders as high as possible and hold for 30 seconds (do two sets of stretches).

4) **Triceps Towel Stretch**

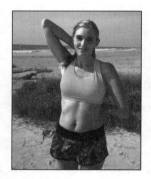

Grab a towel with one hand, and while holding the towel, place your hand behind your head with your fingers touching your head. With your other hand reach behind your back and grasp the other towel end and gently pull to stretch the upper elbow and lateral shoulder muscles.

5) Forearm Rotation Stretch

Grab a broom and raise your elbows so that the humerus (upper arm bones) are parallel to the floor. Hold your elbow position at 90 degrees (making a right angle). Rotate your wrist to being above and behind your head. Hold for 30 seconds before rotating your wrists and the broom down as low as you can move (while still keeping your elbows in a fixed position).

LOWER ARM/WRIST

1) Wrist Rotation

With your arm fully extended, turn your palm outward until your thumb points straight down at the floor. Then retract your arm until your elbow is touching your stomach and again roll your wrist to the outside until your thumb is pointed to the ground.

2) Wrist Flexor Stretch

Stretch the muscle that flexes your hand, making your fingers move closer to your wrist. Place both hands on the wall at chest height. Now slide the hands down a few inches as you lean into the wall. This extreme extension stretches the muscles and tendons on the palm side of the wrist.

3) Wrist Extensor Stretch

Extend your arms and curl one hand downward. Cradle that hand with the other so the second hand's fingers are pointed to the sky. Gently pull on the long hand bones (metacarpals) to stretch the top of your wrist.

HIP/THIGH
1) Supine Knee Tuck

Lay on your back and pull one knee to your chest to stretch your butt and posterior thigh muscles. After the 30 second stretch, repeat the positioning with a more medial (center) alignment or a more lateral alignment.

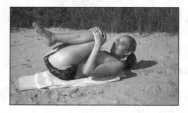

2) Groin Stretch

Sit on your mat and pull your feet to your groin. You can rest your hands on the tips of your toes or on the sides of your ankles. For greater passive stretch, one can also push your knees down with your elbows while leaning over to stretch.

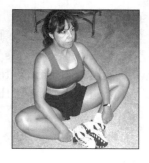

3) Supine Piriformis Stretch

The piriformis muscle attaches the hip bone (femoral head) to the tail bone (sacrum), and tension of this muscle often causes sciatic pain. To stretch, lay on your back with your heels together and then retract one foot to rest upon the other knee. Let the bent knee fold beyond the opposite leg.

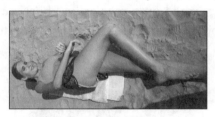

4) Medial & Lateral Quadriceps Stretch

Start by grabbing a firm surface with left hand (or lean on a tall counter or rail) and grab your right ankle. Lean forward and pull your ankle back to stretch the quadriceps (the front muscle on your upper thigh), and hold that stretch for 30 seconds. Then for variation pull your knee away from your body (abduction), which helps stretch different quadriceps muscles.

5) Iliopsoas Stretch

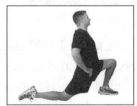

This is like the stretch one would experience from a gentle deep lunge because this muscle attaches the outer hip to the lumbar vertebrae. Stand with your legs 12 inches apart, placing your left leg in front of the right leg. Next, bend your left knee, without letting your feet lose contact with the ground, and lean back to your hip.

Knee
1) Distal Quad Stretch

This is performed on a mat or bed because you lay prone (face down) and pull your heel towards the gluteus muscles.

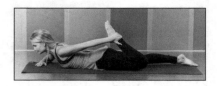

Hamstring Stretching

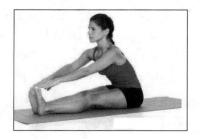

(As described for the lower back) Begin my sitting on the mat with both legs extended, and extend your arms over the legs by bending farther at the waist. This will stretch the hamstrings and maintain a full tension stretch for 30 continuous seconds.

LOWER LEG

1) Calf Towel Stretch

This is a joint-specific passive stretch to increase flexibility in the two heads of the gastrocnemius—calf muscles. Drape a towel across the ball of your foot and pull until it gets tight. Hold each stretch for 30 continuous seconds.

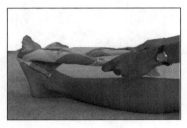

2) Runner's Calf Muscle Stretch

Place one foot in front of the other and lean forward onto a wall. For the first stretch of each foot hold the ankle in a neutral position for 30 seconds before resting 30 seconds by stretching the other calf. Then alternate with an "open" or plie alignment where the heel is closer to the other foot. (Perform each for 30 seconds on each calf) and then use a "closed" position where the ankles are aligned away from the body.

FOOT/ANKLE

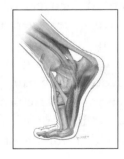

1) Foot Extensors Stretch

To stretch the muscles that make the foot flex (toes up), you can tuck your feet beneath another chair while seated and use a cross bar as resistance to stretch the muscles across the top of your foot. Standing and draping your toes back while leaning forward is also a technique to stretch these muscles.

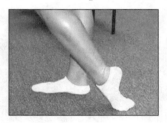

2) Foot Flexors Stretch

Sit in a chair with your foot straight out against the wall. Now keeping contact between the sole of your feet and the wall, slide your foot down the wall until it gets tight. Hold it there for a 30-second stretch.

3) Plantar Fascia Stretch

The plantar fascia is not a longitudinal fiber and the fascia is a pad of connective tissue. This is the source of the #1 most common heel pain (plantar fasciopathy), and the most effective method for treating this pain syndrome is stretching. If you have acute, severe heel pain when you first wake up in the morning, then please see your physician or podiatrist because they can prescribe a stretching device shown effective in reducing the pain (John 2011).

Tools for preventing contracture (shortening and tightening) of the fascia can be done with the towel stretch as described above and with a rolling pin. While seated, simply place the 3" rolling pin beneath one foot and roll forwards and backwards with increasing pressure for 30 seconds (do 2 sets). This will increase the blood flow to the area and reduce the tension in the plantar fascia.

4) Medial/Lateral Stretch

Have your full leg extended on a mat (supine) and rock your foot with your toes pointed towards 3 o'clock while keeping your heel on the mat and hold this for 30 seconds. Then rock your foot to the left towards 9 o'clock and hold for 30 seconds to stretch the lateral and medical connective tissues.

DIGEST THIS

These are the stretches you will need, and they can be used as an Energy Surge if they are challenging enough to raise your heart rate. These stretches are also ideal to give your body a good cool down after aerobic or prolonged resistance training. A stiff, granite body weighs more than a limber rattan reed. Get flexible to stay moving.

13

Exercise-Phys-E-O!

"My loss (40 lb. weight loss and recovery from COPD) was only possible by combining the three easy steps (PEN) from Doc Willis." *(Kim B. from Austin, Texas)*

The physiology of exercise is how the body moves, functions, absorbs oxygen, discards CO_2, pumps blood, responds to physical demands, and burns fat. This can be thought of as exercise medicine because it involves human energy expenditure, human energy transfer, and environmental effects on physiology.

There are three types of contractions that can be used for the muscles:

An **Isometric** contraction is when the muscles are active but no movement is accomplished. It is often called a "static exercise" and if you performed the isometric exercises in Chapter 6, "Easy Exercise," then your groin muscles would activate and tighten, however your legs would not come together. The resistance can be static as if you were holding a ball between your legs or it could be antagonistic if you were simultaneously activating your hip abductor muscles. Both muscles groups were equally activated and the joints did not move.

Isotonic exercises are accomplished with both muscle contraction and joint movement. Isotonic contractions are often used in muscle strength testing such as with a dynamometer. So the force and speed generated in one exercise such as a biceps, barbell curl could be tested simultaneously in an isotonic, dynamometer test.

Isokinetic contractions are most frequently used in rehabilitation, and a dynamometer is used in the case to physically move the joint through the range of motion even though the muscles may be too weak to accomplish this without the equipment. Isokinetic means that the motion is the key component rather than the muscle contraction.

Exercises for Diseases

EXERCISE FOR DEPRESSION has been proven effective. Neurotransmitters are involved in clinical depression, and serotonin deficiencies are thought to be responsible for this disease. That is why the Selective Serotonin Reuptake Inhibitors (SSRI) medication to keep the serotonin levels high is effective, but exercise is always better than medication.

A substantial work was done by Dr. Simon Young (2007) from McGill University in Canada. His work, titled "How to increase serotonin in the human brain without drugs," examined research on four protocols including using positron emission tomography, levels of light, exercise, and diet. The positron emission tomography or PET Scan is not something I would have thought to prescribe for depression, but people reported greater happiness following this procedure when it is used as an experimental treatment.

Daylight's effect on depression has been known for many years and Dr. Young reminded us of the "Light Cafes" in northern UK, Scandinavia, and Austria. They use mirrors to reflex the light into the café which could otherwise be easily blocked by both tall buildings and the mountains. This brings a brighter, happier disposition to people bathe in the sun in these cafes.

I also remembered when I lived outside of Seattle, which is proclaimed to have the largest prescription rate (per capita) of SSRI medication that from January until the summer it is normally overcast and gray. It took three months before I saw a full day of sun and that made a remarkable difference in our mood!

Regarding exercise, the National Health Service in the UK prescribes exercise as the initial treatment for depression. Dr. Young's work described abundant research on serotonin and tryptophan relating to exercise. We know exercise benefits patients with depression and elevates serotonin levels, but now the question is, can exercise effect serotonin levels and how much exercise is needed? A study at the University of Texas at Austin showed that just a single dose of 40-minutes of cardiovascular exercise has an immediate effect on a person's mood.

The National Institute for Health and Clinical Excellence (United Kingdom) said that aerobic exercise significantly increases brain serotonin functions. When one's motor activity increases, the rate serotonin is released within the brain increases which also increases the rate of production of both tryptophan and serotonin. Aerobic exercise increases the mood and serotonin levels so add that to your program if depression is a factor.

We also need to address the effects of diet on depression. Research has also shown that large meals, heavy in proteins also cause serotonin levels to drop. Serotonin is manufactured from tryptophan in the brain. (Tryptophan is also the chemical in turkey that makes one sleepy.) Eating abundant turkey actually lowers the endogenous (on-board) tryptophan levels which also reduces the serotonin. We can't take a serotonin vitamin but eating a small, carbohydrate rich meal will . . . you guessed it . . . raise your serotonin levels. Vitamin B-6 has also been shown to benefit serotonin levels.

EXERCISE FOR HEART DISEASE has abundant evidence how exercise helps strengthen your heart muscle, reduce blood pressure, reduce bad (LDL) cholesterol, increase good (HDL) cholesterol, increase insulin sensitivity, and decrease fatty deposits in your blood vessels that normally cause atherosclerosis. The American Heart Association (AHA) recommends that one performs 30 minutes of moderate-intensity aerobic exercise 5 times per week, (totaling 150 minutes). Or the AHA gives an alternative prescription of 25 minutes in vigorous aerobic exercise 3 days per week plus two bouts of moderate-high intensity resistance training twice a week.

Starting such a schedule overnight would be inadvisable because of secondary risks to micro-trauma injuries and exercise sensation. The American Heart Association also offers encouragement that any exercise is better than none. This level of exercise is more than is required for weight loss and your RightSize program gives you more flexibility than just gym or exercise time.

Exercise for Smoking Cessation has shown significant success and I also offer a Smoking Cessation program that has shown to have 98% success rates. It gradually reduces smoking intake and substituting with cardiovascular (exercise) bursts, along with special drinks and foods. You can see more of this at RightSizeAnyBody.com.

Exercise for Joint Pain sounds backwards but low-intensity exercise and prolonged stretching have been shown to be clinically effective for reducing pain from osteoarthritis to fibromyalgia (intensity and frequency of pain). Using such exercise to increase the endorphin (body high) secretions while also moving the joints through the full range of motions benefits people who suffer from such arthritic pain.

Even the Mayo Clinic starts their recommendation that "Exercise is crucial for people with arthritis." The reasons behind this prescribed treatment includes strengthening the muscles and connective tissues surrounding each joint, and improving bone strength, bone mass density, and one's sleep for restoration of the musculoskeletal system. It helps increase the function at each afflicted joint.

DIGEST THIS

Therapeutic exercise works in treating various injuries and preventing disease. Keep it in mind if you experience any of these conditions.

14

Proof for the Professional

"When I was one of Dr. Willis's students, I looked at the literature which supported his program and took the first step for one PEN once a day. Then after the second step, I lost my first 10 pounds and now I have lost 40 lbs. for a greater self-image and 'Can Do' for any challenge!" *(Amy M, Abilene, Texas)*

This chapter will explore the research that was used in constructing the PEN formula. The first study on the frequency of exercise on fat loss "Frequency of exercise for body fat loss: a controlled, cohort study" (Willis FB, Smith FM, Willis AP, J Strength Cond Res. 2009 Nov. 23 (8):2377-8). The purpose of that study was to examine the changes in body fat mass of previously sedentary, unconditioned subjects who began following the U.S. Surgeon General's recommendation in frequency of exercise. The US Surgeon General's recommendation is to exercise four times per week. Ninety subjects participated in this controlled, cohort study.

The subjects (ages 22-74) in that study all had body fat percentages exceeding 25% of body mass for men and 35% for women. All subjects had not exercised more than once per week in the preceding year, and they all had a fat mass exceeding 40 lbs. (The exact fat mass and changes were measured using a BodPod chamber which measures the exact lean body mass and volume vs. the fat through air displacement plethysmography.)

All subjects were prescribed exercise lasting 30 minutes, four times per week for eight weeks. The exercise prescribed was either 30 minutes of low intensity aerobic exercise (70% Max HR) on exercise in a continuous circuit of 10 selected exercise machines (resistance) for 30 minutes. Participation was tracked after completion of the trial, and the categories were as follows:

Group I: control group accomplished 0-5 days of exercise in 56 days

Group II: exercise only 2 times per week = 15 in 56 days

Group III: exercised 2 to 3 times per week = 16 to 24 of 56 days

Group IV: exercised ≥ 4 times per week ≥ 32 of 56 days

The dependent variable in this study was the change in body fat mass, and the outcomes were categorized on frequency of exercise completed by the subjects. There was significant change in fat loss for all exercise frequencies (2-4 days/week). The only difference between groups that equals the best reduction in fat was the group that followed the prescribed protocol of exercising 4 times per week. This group lost an average of 13 lbs. pure fat (not water or muscle loss) in eight weeks, and that was over a 20% reduction in their fat mass! The body fat mass of the control group who did not exercise actually rose in the eight week trial.

Percentage of Fat Reduction in Trial

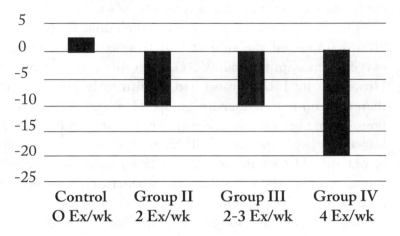

Another significant study in exercise for weight loss was completed by Sijie T1, Hainai Y, Fengying Y, and Jianxiong W. Their study "High intensity interval exercise training in overweight young women" (J Sports Med Phys Fitness. 2012 Jun; 52(3):255-62.) showed that any exercise improved the conditioning of these subjects. Their purpose was to determine if High Intensity Interval Training accomplished significant changes in body composition, cardiac function, and aerobic capacity in overweight young women, ages 19-20.

All of these subjects had BMI ≥ 25 and a percentage of body fat ≥ 30%. The subjects were randomly assigned to one of two groups, the High Intensity Interval Training (HIIT), a High Intensity Continuous Training, or a control group with no exercise training. The difference between HIIT and continuous training is that interval training allows a high and low intensity regime vs a continuous level of exercise. The HIIT group would exercise of intervals at 85% of their max

HR followed by 50% max, followed by 85%, etc. versus the continuous group trained at a constant 50% max level.

This study took 12 weeks for completion. Both exercise groups improved the subjects' BMI, maximum volume of oxygen consumption (max VO2), and other cardiac variables. However, the HIIT group had significantly better results than the continuous exercise group. This study supports the premise that brief levels of elevated heart rate can improve fat loss and other variables. While training continuously at 85% of one max HR would not be safe or advisable for unconditioned or overweight people, it does benefit the overall summation RightSize program.

Dr. Daley led a randomized, controlled trial to determine if therapeutic exercise was beneficial as treatment for psychosocial conditions existing as concurrent pathologies with morbid obesity and the title of this work was "Exercise therapy as a treatment for psychopathologic conditions in obese and morbidly obese adolescents: a randomized, controlled trial" (Daley AJ, Copeland RJ, Wright NP, Roalfe A, Wales JK. Pediatrics. 2006 Nov; 118(5):2126-34.) The study examined 81 adolescent and 18 of 81 were morbidly obese with BMI ≥ 40.

Subjects were randomly assigned to either exercise therapy or a placebo intervention for an eight week duration of one-on-one activity with a therapist followed by a home program for an additional six weeks. The outcome measures were BMI, aerobic fitness and surveys measuring self-perception (physical), self-esteem, and depression. After the total of 14 weeks in one-on-one exercise therapy and home exercise, those subjects did have a significant change in physical self-worth, self-esteem, and depression. There was not a significant change in BMI because of the low variance from the brief 14 week duration. However, if this study had employed the Body Summation score, there could have been significant change in those scores.

The previous two exercise studies were focused on younger subjects but Drs. Eisenmann, Wickel, Welk, and Blair showed the relationship between cardiorespiratory fitness and body fatness during adolescence and cardiovascular disease (CVD) risk factors in adulthood, in "Relationship between adolescent fitness and fatness and cardiovascular disease risk factors in adulthood: the Aerobics Center Longitudinal Study (ACLS)" (J Am pressure 149: 46–53, 2005).

This 11 year longitudinal study of 15 year olds (who matured to 26 years of age) was measured with treadmill time (TM), BMI, percentage body fat, waist circumference, traditional CVD risk factors (blood pressure, fasting total cholesterol, high-density lipoprotein cholesterol [HDL-C], triglycerides [TG], and glucose, and a composite metabolic syndrome risk factor scores were adjusted for age and sex. The results showed a significant relationship between adolescent cardiorespiratory fitness and adult body fatness (obesity), but there was a lack of association between adolescent cardiorespiratory fitness and adult cholesterol, BP, and glucose levels. Adolescent body fatness is correlated to adult cardiovascular disease.

"The effect of a 3-month moderate-intensity physical activity program on body composition in overweight and obese African American college females" was conducted by Drs. Joseph, Casazza, and Durant (Osteoporos Int. 2014 Aug 8). They examined body composition and BMI through a 3-

month study of overweight/obese black women. In this study moderate-intensity aerobic physical activity intervention for overweight and obese young adult women on bone, lean, and fat mass. The average age of the collegiate subjects was 21.7 years of age and their average BMI was 33.3.

The exercise study required participants to engage in four, 30-60-min moderate-intensity aerobic exercise sessions each week. The subjects' BMI was reduced significantly, and this also included reduction of body weight, and increased bone marrow. The exercise prescribed was exactly what is recommended by the US Surgeon General and in RightSize. This exercise regime was effective for collegiate Black women.

"Effects of resistance training frequency on body composition and metabolic and inflammatory markers in overweight postmenopausal women" was a study led by Drs. Orsatti (Lera-Orsatti F, Nahas EA, Maestá N, Nahas Neto J, Lera Orsatti C, Vannucchi Portari G, Burini RC. J Sports Med Phys Fitness. 2014 Jun; 54(3):317-25). This study showed the important outcome of the frequency of resistance training for post-menopausal, sedentary women's body composition and inflammatory markers. The resistance training was similar to the circuit training described in chapter 6, and these women used 60% of their one repetition maximum.

Groups were differentiated on the frequency of exercise participation per week. The greater frequency of training equaled a greater change in weight, but the effect of change in biomarkers of inflammation was independent of frequency. *This suggests that any resistance exercise will benefit women's inflammatory biomarkers for greater outcomes in wellness.*

A capstone work was written by Drs. Blair and Church, "The fitness, obesity, and health equation: is physical activity the common denominator?" (JAMA 292: 1232–1234, 2004).

This was a position paper stating that current research has inadequate links of activity and exercise in the development and reduction of obesity. They examined research that showed correlations in regular exercise and cardiovascular heart disease. In summation they said "regular physical activity has health benefits at any weight, and for those who want or need to lose weight, physical activity is a critical component of long-term weight management."

"Effect of exercise duration and intensity on weight loss in overweight, sedentary women: a randomized trial" was a foundation study by Jakicic et al (JAMA. 2003 Sep 10; 290(10):1323-30.) This study compared intensity of exercise for cardiorespiratory fitness. This study examined 201 women with an average age of 37 and BMI of 32.6 in a 12-month trial. They were randomly assigned to one of four exercise groups: 1) Vigorous intensity/high duration, 2) Moderate intensity/high duration, 3) Moderate intensity/moderate duration, 4) Vigorous intensity/moderate duration.

Significant weight loss was found for all groups and improved cardiorespiratory fitness was seen for all groups. There was not a statistical difference between groups. All subjects lost a mean 16 lbs. (7.5 kg.), and their BMI at the end of the study averaged 29.7. This lets one infer that the frequency of exercise in this controlled study (as found by Willis et al 2009) was a determining variable. The participants exercised four to five times a week, which equals 260 exercise bouts in this 12 month study. It appears that frequency had a greater influence than intensity of exercise.

Nutrition Studies

Organic diets have beneficial effects as shown in a recent study led by Dr. Poulsen.

"Health effect of the New Nordic Diet in adults with increased waist circumference: a 6-mo. randomized controlled trial" (Poulsen SK, Due A, Jordy AB, Kiens B, Stark KD, Stender S, Holst C, Astrup A, Larsen TM., Am J Clin Nutr. 2014 Jan.; 99(1):35-45). This study included 181 obese men and women (age 20-99) with BMI exceeding 30 and an average waist circumference of 40 inches. They were assigned to receive either an organic diet (high in fruit, vegetables, whole grains, and fish) or an average Danish diet for 26 weeks.

The dependent variable was simply change in weight. A total of 147 subjects (81%) completed the intervention, which was home based but included accountability with tracking of all foods supplied these subjects. There was a significant difference for the subjects on the new Danish (organic) diet who had an average 10 lbs. (4.7 kg.) reduction in weight compared to only an average 3 lbs. weight loss by the control group. This also shows that tracking and observance of one's intake can even accomplish weight loss in a rich, traditional, non-organic diet.

The new organic diet also resulted in a significant change in blood pressure as well as waist circumference. These changes were solely caused by change in the quality of products in the subject's diet. There was not a change in exercise or activity, nor in the quantity of food consumed. This is resounding evidence in the benefits of organic, Natural Nutrition, which is one component of the RightSize Formula.

Benefits of organic diets was further elaborated by Wendy

Fries in "The Natural Diet: Best Foods for Weight Loss, You can eat more and still lose weight," which was published in the WebMD website. Her work compiled several different studies and positions of notable nutritional scientist such as Dave Grotto, RD, LDN, who was the author of "101 Foods That Could Save Your Life." They showed that eating "more colors" was beneficial and different from the average American diet that only includes five total pieces of fruit or vegetables a day.

Fries shows that the first secret to *natural foods are that such foods are nutrient dense* compared to starchy foods that are also more readily available for storage as body fat. Her second secret is that *natural foods of fiber provide satiety* so that one feels full after eating compared to carbohydrates such as potato chips, which have been shown to make subjects feel hungrier. The capstone quote is that "Even if you change nothing else in your diet, you're still getting the phytonutrients, chemicals, and as yet unknown nutrients [in produce] that can help protect you from cancer, diabetes, and heart disease," says Christine Gerbstadt, MD, RD, a spokeswoman for the American Dietetic Association.

Organic, natural nutrients are a greater source for one health and RightSize change. While such produce and habits are not for every person at all times, it can be used as one of three components to RightSizing your weight and inches. Wycherley et al proved again that the quality of products being digested results in weight loss.

"Comparison of the effects of weight loss from a high-protein versus standard-protein energy-restricted diet on strength and aerobic capacity in overweight and obese men." (Wycherley TP, Buckley JD, Noakes M, Clifton PM,

Brinkworth GD. Eur J Nutr. 2012 Mar 11), was a study conducted to compare the effects of two low-fat, high protein diets on strength and aerobic capacity measures in overweight and obese men. The two diets differed in the carbohydrate-to-protein ratio, and this was conducted over 12 weeks with 56 men (Age 45 +/- 8).

Subjects were either assigned to a low-fat diet with either High Protein (35%) or a Standard protein (18%), and both diets averaged 7,000 kcal/day. The variables were body weight, body composition, muscle strength, and aerobic capacity. The results were that both groups lost similar amounts of weight (22 vs 19 lbs. in High protein vs. Standard protein), but there was a greater loss of pure fat mass for the High Protein diet vs Standard (17 lbs. vs. 11 lbs.). Both diet benefitted aerobic capacity and the only unique result was the difference in fat mass.

Portion-Size Studies

"Portion control for the treatment of obesity in the primary care setting" was conducted by Kesman et al at the Mayo Clinic (Kesman RL, Ebbert JO, Harris KI, Schroeder DR. (BMC Res Notes. 2011 Sep 9; 4(1):346). Their goal was to evaluate a portion control intervention to facilitate weight loss among obese patients in a primary care setting. The study recruited 65 subjects (40 women and 25 men) who had a BMI from 30 – 40, which is categorized as "obese." The study began with counseling from a dietician and a "Portion Control Plate" for the experimental subjects. The "Portion Plate" was segregated into three sections as follows: ½ for vegetables, ¼ for fish or lean meat, and ¼ for pasta, rice, or whole grains.

The portion plate was to be used for the largest meal of the day (similar to a Pyramid feeding allotment); and for all other meals, they were given a 1 cup bowl. Weights were measured at three and six months. After three months, the portion control group had a significant change in weight of 5 lbs. (2.5 kg.) compared to a 1 lb. loss by the control group. It was curious though that at six months, the change was not any greater in either group. It appears that compliance was an issue because numerous patients reported using the food plate for all meals.

The results showed an attrition rate of 35% and only half of the completed subjects would recommend this protocol to others, which means this was only successful for a one-third of the subjects recruited. Consistency in the portion size or portion quality would be a better protocol as used in the RightSize formula.

Portion size of food affects energy intake in normal weight and overweight men and women was conducted by Rolls, Morris, and Roe (Am J Clin Nutr 2002;76:1207-1213.) and the purpose of this study was to determine if portion control for one meal a day over four weeks will determine the energy outcomes from this alteration. The portion sizes were increased as the study progressed, although the quantity consumed was not controlled. They found that "the ready availability of foods in large portions is likely to be facilitating the overconsumption of energy in many persons." In such cases, these subjects would have better outcomes from fixed portion controls versus quality control.

Dr. Rolls continued this work with a work titled "What is the role of portion control in weight management?" (Int J Obes {Lond}. 2014 Jul; 38) and his paper shows that large portions have a role in development of obesity. As seen in the study by Kesman et al, portion size can be difficult to control, which also supports the three-leg RightSize formula. While portion-control plates have been shown effective in randomized controlled trials on weight loss, less data is available on the long term outcomes from continual portion size controlled eating. Dr. Rolls reminds readers that we need to return to "High-Energy-Dense Foods" (such as organic foods) in appropriate portion sizes.

Drs. Weber and Rose conducted the recent study comparing an internet behavioral weight loss system with commercial portion-controlled foods. "A pilot internet-based behavioral weight loss intervention with or without commercially available portion-controlled foods" (Obesity Silver Spring). 2013 Sep; 21(9):E354-9). Fifty subjects participated (mean age 46 +/- 10 and mean BMI 35.1) and they were randomly assigned to either an internet behavioral weight loss program or that program plus commercially available portion-controlled diet for 12 weeks.

Both groups lost weight. The internet behavioral group lost 10 lbs. and the group which had both internet behavioral counseling plus Portion-controlled diet lost 13 lbs. However, the combined group also showed significant changes in blood pressure, blood glucose, and LDL cholesterol levels. Again the combined programs were of greatest effect, and using a flexible, combined program with different options could be even more effective.

"Body composition, dietary composition, and components of metabolic syndrome in overweight and obese adults after a 12-week trial on dietary treatments focused on portion control, energy density, or glycemic index" was a study conducted by Melanso et al which examined three dietary approaches to weight loss and disease prevention. (Melanson KJ, Summers A, Nguyen V, Brosnahan J, Lowndes J, Angelopoulos TJ, Rippe JM. Nutr J. 2012 Aug 27; 11:57.) Over 12 weeks, sedentary but healthy adults participated in this study and their demographics were as follows: 138 women, 19 men, mean age 39, mean BMI 32.

These subjects attended weekly group sessions for weight loss, combined with either Portion-controlled diet, Low energy density diet, or low glycemic index diet. (Glycemic Index (GI) is a number given to foods and the value is correlated to the effect a food has on one's blood glucose level. The GU represents a person's blood glucose after consuming a food. Peanuts have a GI or 15 compared to French bread = GI of 95.)

All groups in this study showed significant weight loss and change in body composition. Dietary changes were also seen in reduced percentage of fats and increased percentage of proteins, which also helped reduce symptoms of Metabolic Syndrome and reduced HDL values. These scientists agreed in conclusion that flexibility in such programs was more opportune for the subjects' success.

Meal replacement protein rich shakes have been shown effective in short term weight loss studies. Levitsky and Pacanowski examined whether portion size control was responsible for this weight loss in their study "Losing weight without dieting. Use of commercial foods as meal replacements for lunch produces an extended energy deficit" (Appetite. 2011 Oct; 57(2):311-7). Seventeen subjects ate all their meals and snacks from foods provided by their research group from Monday to Friday for five weeks. In the first week, subjects selected food from a buffet where the foods were weighed before eating. Over the next two weeks, half of the group (experimental subjects) chose to eat one of six commercially available portion controlled foods. The controlled foods showed an average 250 kcal reduction per day and the experimental group lost more weight during the portion controlled phase of this study.

"Use of portion-controlled entrees enhances weight loss in women" was a parallel study of women who had BMI scores from 26 to 40. (Hannum SM, Carson L, Evans EM, Canene KA, Petr EL, Bui L, Erdman JW Jr. Obes Res. 2004 Mar; 12(3):538-46.). Sixty women participated (ages 24 to 60), and they were randomly assigned into two groups. The portion-controlled group consumed two frozen entrees daily plus two additional servings from the FDA "Food Group Pyramid." The self-select Diet group were told to consume portions from the Food Group Pyramid (55% carbohydrate, 25% protein, 20% fat) and 1365 kcal. Each group met weekly to monitor compliance and take measures. Outcomes included body weight, composition, hip and waist circumference, blood pressure, fasting blood lipids, glucose, insulin, and C-reactive protein.

The portion-controlled group showed a greater decrease in weight (12.3 lbs.), greater decrease in pure fat mass (8 lbs.), and greater decrease in total cholesterol (24.4 mg./dl). This group had a greater reduction of weight and fat, thereby reducing the risk of cardiovascular disease. These scientists concluded that consuming and accurate, fixed portion size was an effective method in achieving these changes.

Obesity and Health Risks on Earth

Now we will discuss how portion size, exercise, and natural nutrition (PEN) work to eliminate health risks in the United States. Dr. Flegal completed a landmark study with her colleagues who showed the "Association of All-Cause Mortality With Overweight and Obesity Using Standard Body Mass Index Categories" (Flegal KM, Kit BK, Orpana H, Graubard BI. JAMA. 2013 Jan 2; 309(1):71-82). This was a systematic review with meta-analysis, the highest empirical value in clinical research. Instead of examining changes in a certain number of subjects, they examined qualified studies which used BMI as a variable. A sum of 4142 qualified articles were screened, and 97 studies were selected for inclusion to this meta-analysis, which included a total of 2.8 million subjects.

They reviewed why the Body Mass Index based categories are valid boundaries for "Overweight, Preobesity, and Obesity" based on health risks and "Hazard Ratios."

Again the categories are as follows:
1. Underweight (BMI of ≤ 18.5)
2. Normal\weight (BMI of 18.5-25)
3. Overweight (BMI of 26 - 30), and
4. Obesity (BMI of ≥ 30).
   i. Grade 1 obesity, BMI of 30 -34
   ii. Grade 2 obesity, BMI of 35 – 39
   iii. Grade 3 obesity, BMI ≥ 40

Their conclusion from this amazing body of evidence was that "Relative to normal weight, obesity (all grades) and grades 2 and 3 obesity were both associated with significantly higher all-cause mortality. Grade 1 obesity was not associated with higher mortality, suggesting that the excess mortality in obesity may predominantly be due to elevated mortality at higher BMI levels." They said that the Overweight category had a lower Health Risk Ratio but was still relevantly higher than the Normal weight BMI category.

In a more specified study, Dr. Hu showed evidence in "Overweight and Obesity in Women: Health Risks and Consequences. (J Womens Health 12: 163–172, 2003). Dr. Hu stated that

> "… the adverse effects of obesity on women's health is overwhelming and indisputable. Obesity, especially abdominal obesity, is central to the metabolic syndrome and is strongly related to polycystic ovary syndrome (PCOS) in women. Obese women are particularly susceptible to diabetes, and diabetes, in turn, puts women at dramatically increased risk of cardiovascular disease (CVD). Obesity substantially increases the risk of several major cancers in women, especially postmenopausal breast cancer and endometrial cancer."

The risks Dr. Hu showed as directly correlated for women with obesity include the following: Blood pressure, Blood lipids, Insulin Resistance (Type II Diabetes), Cholelethiasis, Polycystic Ovarian Syndrome, Metabolic Syndrome, Thrombogenic (plasma/fibrogen) Factors, and Systemic Inflammation. In summation Dr. Hu said,

> "Obesity is a complex problem resulting from a com-

bination of genetic, behavioral, environmental, cultural, and socioeconomic influences. However, behavioral and environmental factors are primary determinants of obesity, and lifestyle modification has been shown to be extremely effective in preventing type 2 diabetes through moderate weight loss. Because most Americans do not engage in regular physical activity (especially women) or follow a healthy eating pattern, the task of reversing the obesity trend is an enormous challenge, which calls for changes not only in diet and lifestyle at individual levels but also in policy, physical and social environment, and cultural norms."

CDC Findings (from Dr. Willis's class on 'Fitness for Living' 2012):

As of 2014, 67% of the US population are categorized as "Overweight," which includes inactivity which is a clinical condition detrimental to one's health. The US Center for Disease Control (CDC) has shown that most of the top causes of death are preventable, avoidable, or curable through behavior, exercise, and lifestyle. The United States is only 33rd of 193 in life-expectancy, and while we pride ourselves on our health care system, we are not effective in preventive medicine with exercise.

The country with the greatest life expectancy is Japan (mean life of 83 years), and they also have the lowest incidence of obesity (3% compared to 33% in the USA). Since the 1960s, obesity incidence has doubled in the USA. What is the cause of such a drastic increase, and what are we doing to change this disease?

In 2008 the US Surgeon General reported that 7 of 10 American deaths were due to "preventable chronic diseases" such as Cardiovascular Heart Disease, Type II Diabetes, and Chronic Obstructive Pulmonary Disease (COPD) from smoking. The American College of Sports Medicine and the American Heart Association have recommended the following for healthy adults age 18 to 65:

• Moderate intensity aerobic physical activity for a minimum of 30 minutes, four days a week or vigorous intensity aerobic physical activity for a minimum of 20 minutes three days a week. (That means just the time of one movie each week needs to be dedicated to exercise.)

• Activities that maintain or increase muscular strength and endurance a minimum of two days per week on nonconsecutive days.

Those directions were made in 2007 and are simple, but why have they not been successful? The answer is that it is a more complex lifestyle change than just increasing activity alone. Of course we all should be more active, but with the right formula, a successful in a lifelong change is possible. What exercise is the optimal exercise for fat loss? Exercise has many benefits beyond decreased fat mass, such as increased bone density, decreased blood pressure, decreased cholesterol, and decreased depression or anxiety.

This book combines the appropriate aerobic and anaerobic exercise with quality, natural, nutritional foods, and portion size control in a personalized plan that accomplishes a permanent change in one's physique, wellness, and fitness!

Our bodies were made to move and must move in order to maintain healthy and normal function Research has shown conclusive and direct correlations, showing that appropriate exercise benefits or prevents the following conditions:

CARDIOVASCULAR HEART DISEASE
- Myocardial Infarction
- Atherosclerosis
- Hypertension
- Hyperlipidemia
- High Cholesterol
- Varicose veins

DIABETES MELLITUS
- Insulin Sensitivity (Type II)

OSTEOARTHRITIS

CANCER

SLEEP DISORDERS

DEPRESSION

Exercise prescriptions vary with frequency, intensity, and time or duration (FIT). The acronym FIT can be used to show the difference between aerobic threshold training versus anaerobic or resistance training. The goals of aerobic versus anaerobic exercise are different so the same exercise and resistance can be altered with FIT to accommodate the personal needs and goals of each patient.

Frequency can refer to the number of total exercise sessions, the number of sets of exercise or the individual repetitions during a particular exercise. Intensity is the workload, resistance, perceived exertion or Heart Rate (HR) employed during the exercise routine. The time, or duration, can mean the total time for an exercise session or the duration of one set. Aerobic threshold training is training with the optimal volume of oxygen consumption (VO2). Aerobic threshold training consumes body fat as fuel versus anaerobic training, which uses glucose as the primary fuel source.

AEROBIC EXERCISE affects the following:
• Insulin sensitivity
• High blood pressure
• Hyperlipidemia (high cholesterol)
• Respiratory disorders such as COPD
• Atherosclerosis
    (fatty occlusions blocking coronary arteries)
• Arteriosclerosis (hardening of the arteries)
• Reduces depression

ANAEROBIC EXERCISE can accomplish the following:
• Injury prevention
• Increased basal metabolic rate
• Increased Bone Mass Density (osteoporosis)
• Increased muscularity & strength for greater function
• Joint injury recuperation
• Prevents and reduces arthritis
• Reducing blood glucose and beneficial in reducing
    prediabetic conditions

Exercise can also be very beneficial for special groups such as the elderly and women in maternity. People of advanced age experience reduction in the ventilatory perfusion

(VQ), which is the effective transfer of blood and oxygen in the lungs. Estimates are that the VQ drops 5-10% each year from age 40–80 years of age; and low intensity, progressive aerobic endurance training can restore and improved the oxygen transfer.

Exercise has been shown effective in pregnancy with benefits for both the mother and child. The appropriate prescribed exercise benefits the mother's conditioning for reduced intensity and shorter durations during labor with reduced fat retention, reduced postpartum depression, and faster recovery post-delivery. For the child, maternal exercise has shown improved organ development, improved stress tolerance, and advanced neurobehavioral maturation with testing at five years.

Type II Diabetes Mellitus is a growing, preventable, and curable pathology. Prescribed exercise has shown to result in increased insulin sensitivity and more stable blood glucose levels as seen in HbA1c testing. Exercise has "cured" this condition in some of my clients who have been taken off all oral medication. This has saved the patients from experiencing the secondary pathologies such as heart attack, glaucoma, and peripheral neuropathy yielding uncontrollable open wound infections and non-traumatic amputations.

According to the CDC, the Top 10 Causes of Death in the Unites States are Cardiovascular Heart Disease (CHD), Cancer, Chronic Obstructive Pulmonary Disease (COPD), Cerebrovascular accident or stroke (CVA), accidents, Alzheimer's disease, Diabetes Mellitus, influenza/ pneumonia, nephritis (autoimmune), and suicide. Half of these are controllable and avoidable diseases with the right formula of natural nutrition, portion-size, and exercise.

Figure 1. Atherosclerosis

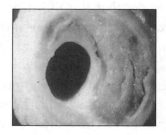

Figure 2. Fatty Heart

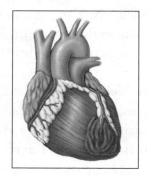

Prevention of treatment for Cardiovascular Heart Disease is easily obtainable through portion size controls, low intensity exercise, and nutrition PEN). The top rule for reducing onset of CHD is "BBC" which means to keep blood pressure, blood glucose, and cholesterol under control. This is easily achieved through the protocols in this book.

• First, don't smoke, or start a smoking cessation program if you do. (Using specific Cardiac Pump exercise intervals to reduce cravings for nicotine has been proven effective.)

• Eat low-fat meals that are rich in fruits and vegetables. (See chapters 7, 8, 15, 17.)

• Eat fish twice a week and take vitamin supplements of Omega-3—Linoleic fatty acid. (The good fat carries away the bad fat.)

• Exercise every other day. (Low-moderate intensity aerobic training and endurance resistance training)

• Drink 2-4 cups of red wine each week (in separate, single consumptions).

Obesity and being overweight are pandemic states of disease in our country. These people are simply suffering from pathology, and this book will empower them to design a unique, effective, and enjoyable program for permanent weight loss and lifestyle retention. We are all different, so each protocol for weight and fat loss must be unique and personalized. In most cases it was not medication or surgery that caused a person to become overweight or obese, yet why is it that we look to those choices for resolution of this lifestyle pathology? Let's use the simplest solution of Portion control, Exercise, and Natural nutrition to return our country to the top life expectancy and the lowest in obesity! Are you ready to take the necessary steps towards change?

DIGEST THIS

This is the proven research that your clinicians will learn about at their next national conference on rehabilitation and/or weight loss. These studies give irrefutable proof of the benefits from the RightSize PEN program.

15

Top Steps

"After giving birth to my son, I was sad, sedentary, and chemically depressed. Instead of taking medicine, I started Doc's program and he helped me lose the depression...and 20 pounds!" (Dr. Amy W., St. Maarten, has maintained her RightSize for five years)

1. First thing in the morning after you awake, start the day with an Energy Surge exercise (immediately and with scissor kicks you don't even have to get out of bed!) This will raise your heart rate and your metabolism. You can also do the floor to ceiling jumps. A friend who is in a wheelchair simply shakes two cans of organic beans (16 oz.) as fast as he can for 100 seconds. (After he got married, his new bride was curious why he had two cans of beans bedside, but she is now a can shaker too!)

2. After you exercise, eat one small bite of a low glycemic index food like a strawberry. Even one bite of a donut is better than keeping your metabolism asleep. Tease your body with this taste and "Forecast your food" for a day of elevated metabolism.

3. Quickly drink a 2-cup portion of pure water. This tells your body that you will stay hydrated throughout the day, and then consume ½ liter of water throughout the day which helps the chemical reactions for consumption of foods digested and body fat onboard.

4. Avoid diet sodas and artificially flavored foods.

5. Put your bathroom scale in the closet or the attic. You only need it for your Body Summation once a month.

6. Eat 5-6 meals a day (every two to three hours) to keep your metabolic fire high.

7. Use Energy Surge exercise before at least two of those six meals. Combining two portions of P+E+N (Portion-size + Energy Surge) will make an even greater elevation of your metabolism for amazing results.

8. Digest at least two meals of Natural foods each day.

9. Make love with your spouse 3-4 times a week. The fifteen minute routines are fine, but making it a two-hour event is much better than watching a movie! Ladies, please support me in this. It is not the final move but the slow, building, sensual meal that builds to rapture, right?

10. Stop eating 10-12 hours before your planned wake up time. (Stop eating three hours before bed plus eight hours needed sleep = 11 hours.) This fast is needed to eliminate any chemicals ingested and restore fluids and minerals to the cells.

11. Every day for two minutes sit alone in a quiet place and say to yourself, "Champion, healthy, and beautiful." Then repeatedly say "Can do!" As you say it and "see it," then your

victory becomes reality. You get what you see and plan for, so instead of saying, "Oh I will always be big," change your words and your vision to say, "I'm starting my RightSize program and I WILL reduce my body size, improve my health, and live a longer, more energetic life! "Believe that you have already received it, and it will be yours!" (Mark 11:24)

12. Plan your success (PEN) to reach the victory tomorrow, and you will be a victor not a victim. You need to push aside any nonbelievers who pull you down. Call and talk to a RightSize mentor who was in your shoes and had as many challenges as you have *(see info at back of book)*. You are not alone and you are on the team of Champions!

In summation, if you combine all these top steps by eating six meals/day (1.5 cup portions) of natural foods and performing an Energy Surge exercise six times a day, then you should have guaranteed results unless you have untreated metabolic or endocrine pathologies. The best part of this program, though, is that you have flexibility for different events and situations. Always try to eat six meals a day with portion size, or eat natural foods only three times a day with Energy Surge before three other meals, and you will have victory in your success! (1 Cor. 15:57)

These top steps can be adapted. While the Energy Surge is vital, it can be adapted if one is taking a beta-blocker medication such as Propranolol. The nutritional values can be changed if someone has diabetes. (Never say you "are diabetic" because it is just an illness. When you have the sniffles you don't say, "I am the flu!") Adaptations, modification, and flexibility can be done by your RightSize coaches. Check us out at www.docwillis.org to see our full team!

DIGEST THIS

This chapter discussed frequency of steps that include performing at least three of the 2-3 minute Energy Surge routines each day and eating 5-6 times a day, making love to your spouse several times a week, stop eating 11 hours before you wake up, and giving yourself "private time" just a few minutes a day. This helps speed up your digestion, wellness, and empower your RightSize for a lifetime!

16

Scripture

"It is easy to hit road blocks or plateaus but what always helped encourage, empower and inspire my progress along any pathway is the Word."

God wants us to have abundant wellness!

Forgetting what is behind and straining toward what is ahead, I press on toward the goal to win the prize for which God has called me heavenward in Christ Jesus (Phil. 3:13-14).

Do you not know that your bodies are temples of the Holy Spirit, who is in you, whom you have received from God? You are not your own (1 Cor. 6:19).

Jesus looked at them and said, "With man this is impossible, but with God all things are possible" (Matt. 19:26).

For the word of God will never fail (Luke 1:37).

Jesus looked at them intently and said, "Humanly speaking, it is impossible. But not with God. Everything is possible with God" (Mark 10:27 NLT).

I know that our Abba Father wants us to be well, joyous, and celebrating life! We failed when He gave us everything (the Garden of Eden), but He gave us a second chance in Jesus Christ and the Holy Spirit! Let's boldly proclaim that we will be as God meant us to be, physically as well!

What does God say to our challenges?

What, then, shall we say in response to these things? If God is for us, who can be against us? (Rom. 8:31)

Don't you realize that in a race everyone runs, but only one person gets the prize? So run to win! (1 Cor. 9:24 NLT)

So whether you eat or drink or whatever you do, do it all for the glory of God (1 Cor. 10:31).

For the LORD your God has blessed you in all that you have done; He has known your wanderings through this great wilderness. These forty years the LORD your God has been with you; you have not lacked a thing (Deut. 2:7 NASB).

My son, do not forget my teaching, but keep my commands in your heart, for they will prolong your life many years and bring you peace and prosperity. Let love and faithfulness never leave you; bind them around your neck, write them on the tablet of your heart. Then you will win favor and a good name in the sight of God and man. Trust in the LORD with all your heart and lean not on your own understanding; in all your ways submit to him, and he will make your paths straight. Do not be wise in your own eyes; fear the LORD and shun evil. This will bring health to your body and nourishment to your bones (Prov. 3:1-8).

God gives us the "Can do" attitude! Let's use it to glorify Him and celebrate our salvation by obtaining our RightSize! I will stand by you proudly as we tell the world that it is God who brought you back or took you to a different, healthier place in your shell that looks more like your forever essence in our human eyes!

Let's build each other up!

To equip his people for works of service, so that the body of Christ may be built up until we all reach unity in the faith and in the knowledge of the Son of God and become mature, attaining to the whole measure of the fullness of Christ (Eph. 4:12-13).

I say to the LORD, "You are my Lord; apart from you I have no good thing" (Psalm 16:2).

Delight yourself in the LORD; And He will give you the desires of your heart (Psalm 37:4 NASB).

I can do all this through him who gives me strength (Phil. 4:13).

You have read the success stories and you know that I want to be your cheerleader, coach, and partner in obtaining your goals! Then we'll set even higher goals that you will reach even more easily! Let your story be an "!" (exclamation mark).

Believe what God wants for you!

This is the confidence we have in approaching God: that if we ask anything according to his will, he hears us. 15 And if we know that he hears us—whatever we ask—we know that we have what we asked of him (1 John 5:14-15).

Therefore I tell you, whatever you ask for in prayer, believe that you have received it, and it will be yours (Mark 11:24).

Then he said to Thomas, "Put your finger here; see my hands. Reach out your hand and put it into my side. Stop doubting and believe!" (John 20:27)

Thanks be to God! He gives us the victory through our Lord Jesus Christ (1 Cor. 15:57).

The LORD himself goes before you and will be with you; he will never leave you nor forsake you. Do not be afraid; do not be discouraged (Deut. 31:8).

Therefore, if anyone is in Christ, the new creation has come:[a] The old has gone, the new is here! (2 Cor. 5:17).

Trust in the Lord!

May he give you the desire of your heart and make all your plans succeed. May we shout for joy over your victory and lift up our banners in the name of our God. May the LORD grant all your requests (Psalm 20:4-5).

"He trusts in the Lord," they say, "let the Lord rescue him. Let him deliver him, since he delights in him" (Psalm 22:8).

The Lord is my strength and my shield; my heart trusts in him, and he helps me. My heart leaps for joy, and with my song I praise him (Psalm 28:7).

Trust in the Lord and do good; dwell in the land and enjoy safe pasture (Psalm 37:3).

Trust in the LORD and do good; dwell in the land and enjoy safe pasture. Take delight in the LORD, and he will give you the desires of your heart. Commit your way to the LORD; trust in him and he will do this; He will make your righteous reward shine like the dawn, your vindication like the noonday sun (Psalm 37:3-6).

You turned my wailing into dancing; you removed my sackcloth and clothed me with joy, that my heart may sing your praises and not be silent. LORD my God, I will praise you forever (Psalm 30:11-12).

Do you believe? Whitney Houston and Mariah Carey sing that when you believe, you will accomplish what you need to. There can be miracles when you believe!

Do you believe?! You have faith in salvation, so also have a mustard seed of faith in your *RightSize!* Do you believe?!

DIGEST THIS

God wants the very best for us, including our RightSize physique.

17

Support for Success

"I previously smoked and when I tried to stop, I would balloon up by 20 pounds. Then I tried Doc's PEN program, and I quit letting food make me overweight. He coached me in smoking cessation as he saved my heart and my bikini!" *(Germain A., Dallas, Texas)*

Gain support from me and my team. We will provide coaching and support by ACSM certified personal trainers, exercise physiologists, and physiotherapists. Now that you have ready this simple, easy, flexible, three option program, we give you assurance that you can accomplish these steps to reach your goal. Boldly say out loud "Can do!" You can contact coaches, cheerleaders, and me at www.DocWillis.org

Sample Programs

The following is a sample program for everyday which is quite often what I consume when I am working at the Shriner's Hospitals for Children.

Work Day Food

• Wake up and before getting out of bed, perform 120 scissor kicks in two minutes! (That is your first brief, brisk exercise of the day as described in Chapter 6.) Then immediately eat one small bite of low glycemic food like one strawberry (not a sugar or starch) to raise your metabolism and drink 2 cups of water to start your day hydrated. (I also like to add a chewable Vitamin C.)

• 7 am Short 20-30 minute bicycle ride followed by the following: half bagel and half apple with a glass of orange juice, (cream cheese is fine because unless the bagel is homemade, this is an Exercise or Portion meal)

The short bicycle ride is good for your metabolism, heart, lungs, but it may also help clear your mind!

• 9 am CLIFF Builder's protein bar + natural lemon lime soda (Portion)

• 11:30 am Run up four flights of stairs and then eat one serving at hospital cafeteria: fried chicken breast, green beans, and mashed potatoes. (Brief Exercise #2)

• 2 pm One orange or grapefruit (Natural) and occasionally I will have an organic pop-tart.

• 4:30 My sweetie and I often go out to eat in the evening, and we'll split a pulled-pork sandwich with homemade chips and one beer. (Portion)

• 7 pm If you are hungry before bed, then grab one string cheese stick or one bite of baked Crock Pot chicken (1 oz.) more than 3 hours before bedtime.

Cruise Food

We enjoy cruising and here is a sample dining plan that I used and lost five pounds with on a 5-day Carnival Cruise!

• 7:00 am Perform 50 Floor to Ceiling Jumps (where you touch the floor and immediately jump to touch the ceiling and repeat 50 times without stopping.) Quickly drink two cups of water and eat a quick bite of fruit as we celebrate sunrise with a mimosa! (Portion)

• 9:00 am Breakfast in the formal dining where we enjoyed splitting huevos rancheros, poached eggs with black beans and cheese. Coffee and cream plus water (Portion size)

• 11:30 am Fish and chips following a brisk charge up all the stairs to the putt-putt golf, activities deck (Exercise and Portion)

• 2:00 pm Fruit & snacks (Natural and Portion) while we played the Gender Competition games (male vs female) with rum punch for the victors!

• 6:00 pm Formal, black-tie dinner with succulent grilled fish topped with crab and capers! (Portion). On another day I chose to have "only cake" for dinner (Portion)!

• 8:00 pm We each had a scrumptious dessert, and mine was the Chocolate Decadence cake, which was an all organic celebration! (I lost a pound that day!)

A Christmas/Football Feast

This is a cultural event in the US, but this can also be used to raise one's metabolism and effectively make it a meal to reduce one's size!

• 8 am Start with Scissor Kicks in bed and then eat a

quick bite of fruit (one strawberry). Then briskly walk your dog around the block before opening Christmas presents. (Exercises #1 and 2)

• 8:30 am   Family Brunch of waffles, bacon, and fruit with orange juice! (Natural because it was all organic products for the pastry and protein, and all natural fresh fruits)

• 12:30 pm   On the way to the noon football game, we each ate a Breakfast Taco at a local fast food restaurant just to keep our metabolism high. (Portion)

• 2:30 pm   At halftime the whole family did "Floor to Ceiling" jumps as competition to see who got the last pie of Dutch Apple Pie! Then we ate hamburgers only (we skipped the fries) so we could enjoy the right size of huge juicy, homemade burgers that would alone would fill a cereal bowl (1.5 cups if blended to a liquid). (Exercise #3 plus Portion)

Okay, I admit to previously putting one of these burgers in a blender to see how much was the right amount (1.5 cups portion size).

• 4:30 pm   Fruit and nuts after we briefly chased the kids in the parking lot after the game (Brief Exercise #4)

• 7:30 pm   We had fajita tacos on the way home. One huge taco plus a few chips with fresh salsa equaled the right size (Portion).

• If we are staying up late, then we force ourselves to eat a piece of fruit three hours before bedtime. (Natural).

Keeping Your RightSize Forever

After you finish this program, will you ever have weight issues again? Weight issues may come again, but they can be even more easily overcome. RightSize works in any situation.

When I was a professor in west Texas I had chronic sinus infections (sinusitis) because I was so allergic to the environment. I gained 30 pounds because I was sick 9 of 12 months. However, as soon as I was free of the infections, I started my RightSize program and lost over 45 lbs. to regain my right size of 180 lbs. It was easy and after I did my food forecasting, I simply just used Energy Surge exercise bouts when I was not able to eat natural foods. (I never eat more than 1.5 cups because I eat 5-6 times a day.) There are things that may happen to cause temporary weight gain, but we can use this formula to make our wellness and size right!

Metabolism Tips:

1) The Energy Surge exercise for 2-3 minutes will always raise your metabolism, and with scissor kicks you can start as soon as you wake up! You don't need to get dressed and go to the gym; rev up your metabolism from your first minute of being awake! Remember the little kids running in the playground? If you could do five of 2-3 minute Energy Surge exercise bouts a day, that might be all you need to achieve your RightSize. (Remember that is what our victory model CJ did.) However, if you are at a banquet with the President, you may not want to run around the table 10 times before you eat! LOL! In that situation, just eat a Portion size.

2) Eating more often but in smaller portions has been shown in numerous studies to keep your metabolism high and reduce fat! If you eat Portion-size, then it has to be all day long. Forecast your food and plan to eat like the person you choose to see in the mirror!

3) Eating natural foods (organic when possible) will al-

ways raise your metabolism. Combine the protocols, and that is an acceleration plan that several of our victors have used to overcome a plateau.

4) Starting the morning with one tease bite of food before you exercise will also raise your metabolism from the night's fast. One strawberry and the quick Energy Surge exercise bout will skyrocket your metabolism even if you are not choosing to do your cardio or resistance exercise routine today.

5) Use the fuel analogy and use a low flame to gain our RightSize and show the world that we can beat any challenge with sustained, prolonged, low intensity efforts.

6) Be positive, even if you don't want to! Every day for two minutes sit alone in a quiet place and remind yourself of your positive attributes and that you can do it. As you say it and see it, then your victory will become reality. (Read, pray, and believe the words of Jesus in Mark 11:24.)

7) Forecast your food and plan your PEN for success today!

8) You can do more Energy Surge exercise bouts each day besides just before you eat. Why not?

Let's go back to the fuel analogy. The small fire will burn continuously with small inputs of wood (fuel). If we throw too much fuel on, the burn will be less efficient (lots of ash and unburned wood that has to be disposed of). If we have fuel with no pilot light (no exercise), then we could have major damage like with the explosion beneath a big hot water heater.

Together let's lose 100 million pounds this year! How much will you contribute to that goal? After you gain your

RightSize, who will you recruit to join you in this righteous victory? Would you be a positive, empowering coach to others? Let's say it together, "Can do!" Say it more loudly because you know and believe that the flexible PEN tools will work. Let me ask if you will achieve your RightSize, and say it with me ... "Can do!" Amen!

DIGEST THIS

These samples show how you can use PEN individually or together to keep your metabolism high throughout the day and consume more body fat as fuel rather than storing more! At the Christmas feast we ate lots of food but in the right portion size or all natural for faster digestion, and we completed four brief exercise bouts without ever breaking a sweat!

Use PEN to write your success and share your success as a RightSize Victor!

Bibliography

1. Willis FB, Smith FM, Willis AP. **Frequency of exercise for body fat loss: a controlled, cohort study.** *J Strength Cond Res.* 2009 Nov. 23; (8):2377-80.

2. Wycherley TP, Buckley JD, Noakes M, Clifton PM, Brinkworth GD. **Comparison of the effects of weight loss from a high-protein versus standard-protein energy-restricted diet on strength and aerobic capacity in overweight and obese men.** *Eur J Nutr.* 2012 Mar. 11.

3. Kesman RL, Ebbert JO, Harris KI, Schroeder DR. **Portion control for the treatment of obesity in the primary care setting.** *BMC Res Notes.* 2011 Sep. 9; 4(1):346.

4. Batsis, JA, Romero-Corral, A, Collazo-Clavell, ML, Sarr, MG, Somers, VK, Brekke, L, and Lopez-Jimenez, F. **Effect of weight loss on predicted cardiovascular risk: change in cardiac risk after bariatric surgery.** *Obesity* 15: 772–784, 2007.

5. Sijie T, Hainai Y, Fengying Y, Jianxiong W. **High intensity interval exercise training in overweight young women.** *J Sports Med. Phys. Fitness.* 2012 Jun; 52(3):255-62.

6. Blair, SN and Church, TS. **The fitness, obesity, and health equation: is physical activity the common denominator?** *JAMA* 292: 1232–1234, 2004.

7. Daley, AJ, Copeland, RJ, Wright, NP, Roalfe, A, and Wales, JK. **Exercise therapy as a treatment for psychopathologic conditions in obese and morbidly obese adolescents: a randomized, controlled trial.** *Pediatrics* 118: 2126–2134, 2006.

8. Davis, JA, Dorado, S, Keays, KA, Reigel, KA, Valencia, KS, and Pham, PH. **Reliability and validity of the lung volume measurement made by the BOD POD body composition system.** *Clin Physiol Funct. Imaging* 27: 42–46, 2007.

9. Eisenmann, JC, Wickel, EE, Welk, GJ, and Blair, SN. **Relationship between adolescent fitness and fatness and cardiovascular disease risk factors in adulthood: the Aerobics Center**

Longitudinal Study (ACLS). *Am pressure* J 149: 46–53, 2005.

10. Ginde, SR, Geliebter, A, Rubianof, A, Silva, AM,Wang, J, Heshka, S, Heymsfield, SB. **Air displacement plethysmography: validation in overweight and obese subjects.** *Obes. Res.* 13: 1232–1237, 2005.

11. Hu, FB. **Overweight and Obesity in Women: Health Risks and Consequences.** *J Womens Health* 12: 163–172, 2003.

12. Irwin, ML, Yasui, Y, Ulrich, CM, Bowen, D, Rudolph, RE, Schwartz, RS, Yukawa, M, Aiello, E, Potter, JD, and Mctiernan, A. **Effect of exercise on total and intra-abdominal body fat in post-menopausal women: a randomized controlled trial.** *JAMA* 289:323–330, 2003.

13. Jakicic, JM, Marcus, BH, Gallagher, KI, Napolitano, M, and Lang,W. **Effect of exercise duration and intensity on weight loss in overweight, sedentary women: a randomized trial.** *JAMA.* 290: 1323–1330, 2003.

14. Jahicic, JM and Otto, AD. **Treatment and prevention of obesity: what is the role of exercise?** *Nutr. Rev.* 64: S57–S61, 2006.

15. Kraemer, WJ, Torine, JC, Silvestre, R, French, DN, Ratamess, NA, Spiering, BA, Hatfield, DL, Vingren, JL, and Volek, JS. **Body size and composition of National Football League players.** *J Strength Cond. Res.* 19: 485–489, 2005.

16. Mccullough, PA,Gallagher,MJ, Dejong, AT, Sandberg, KR, Trivax, JE, Alexander, D, Kasturi, G, Jafri, SM, Krause, KR, Chengelis, DL, Moy, J, and Franklin, BA. **Cardiorespiratory fitness and short-term complications after bariatric surgery.** *Chest* 130: 517–525, 2006.

17. Minderico, CS, Silva, AM, Teixeira, PJ, Sardinha, LB, Hull, HR, and Fields, DA. **Validity of air-displacement plethys-mography in the assessment of body composition changes in a 16-month weight loss program.** *Nutr. Metab.* (Lond) 3: 32, 2006.

18. Moras, A, Lee, I, Buring, JE, and Ridker, PM. **Association of physical activity and body mass index with novel and traditional**

cardiovascular biomarkers in women. *JAMA* 295: 1412–1419, 2006.

19. Noreen, EE and Lemon, PW. **Reliability of air displacement plethysmography in a large, heterogeneous sample.** *Med. Sc.i Sports Exerc.* 38: 1505-1509, 2006.

20) Pescatello, LS. **Exercise and hypertension: recent advances in exercise prescription.** *Curr. Hypertens. Rep.* 7: 281–286, 2005.

21. Shaw, I and Shaw, BS. **Consequences of resistance training on body composition and coronary artery disease risk.** *Cardio. J So. Africa* 17: 111–116, 2006.

22. Tucker, La and Peterson, Tr. **Objectively measured intensity of physical activity and adiposity in middle-aged women.** *Obes. Res.* 11: 1581–1587, 2003.

23. Voelker, R. **Studies suggest dog walking a good strategy for fostering fitness.** *JAMA* 296: 643, 2006.

24. Volaklis, KA, Douda, HT, Kokkino, PF, and Tokmakidis, SP. **Physiological alterations to detraining following prolonged combined strength and aerobic training in cardiac patients.** *Eur. J Cardiovasc. Prev. Rehabil.* 13: 375–380, 2006.

25. Warburton, DE, Nicol, CW, and Bredin, SS. **Health benefits of physical activity: the evidence.** *CMAJ* 174: 801–809, 2006.

26. Wessel, TR, Arant, CB, Olson, MB, Johnson, BD, Reis, SE, Sharaf, BL, Shaw, LJ, Handberg, E, Sopko, G, Kelsey, SF, Pepine, CJ, and Merz, NB. **Relationship of physical fitness vs body mass index with coronary artery disease and cardiovascular events in women.** *JAMA* 292: 1179–1187, 2004.

27. Farrell SW, Braun L, Barlow CE, Cheng YJ, Blair SN. **The relation of body mass index, cardiorespiratory fitness, and all-cause mortality in women.** *Obes. Res.* 2002 Jun. 10(6):417-23.

28. Kreiger JW. **Single vs. multiple sets of resistance exercise for muscle hypertrophy: a meta-analysis.** *J Strength Cond. Res.* 2010 Apr. 24(4):1150-9.

29. Dickinson JM, Rasmussen BB. Amino acid transporters in

the regulation of human skeletal muscle protein metabolism. *Curr. Opin. Clin. Nutr. Metab. Care.* 2013 Nov. 16(6):638-44.

30. Wang J, Vanegas SM, Du X, Noble T, Zingg JM, Meydani M, Meydani SN, Wu D. **Caloric restriction favorably impacts metabolic and immune/inflammatory profiles in obese mice but curcumin/piperine consumption adds no further benefit.** *Nutr. Metab.* (Lond). 2013 Mar 27; 10(1):29. doi: 10.1186/1743-7075-10-29.

31. Rolls BJ, Morris EL, Roe LS. **Portion size of food affects energy intake in normal-weight and overweight men and women.** *Am. J Clin. Nutr.* 2002. 76:1207-1213.

32. Stienstra R, Duval C, Müller M, Kersten S. PPARs, **Obesity, and Inflammation.** *PPAR Res.* 2007. 2007:95974.

33. Berardi, J. *The Metabolism Advantage,* Rodale Press, 2006.

34. Benardot D. **Timing of Energy and Fluid Intake: New Concepts for Weight Control and Hydration.** *ACSM Health & Fitness Journal.* 2007. 11(4):13-19.

35. Deutz B, Benardot D, Martin D, and Cody M. **Relationship between energy deficits and body composition in elite female gymnasts and runners.** *Medicine & Science in Sports & Exercise.* 2000; 32(3): 659-668.

36. Iwao, S., K. Mori, and Y. Sato. **Effects of meal frequency on body composition during weight control in boxers.** *Scandinavian Journal of Medicine & Science in Sports.* 6(5):265Y272, 1996.

37. Bell SJ, Van Ausdal W, Grochoski G **Do dietary supplements help promote weight loss?** *J Diet Suppl.* 2009. 6(1):33-53.

38. Pan A, Yu D, Demark-Wahnefried W, Franco OH, Lin X. **Meta-analysis of the effects of flaxseed interventions on blood lipids,** *Am. J Clin. Nutr.* 2009 Aug. 90(2): 288-97.

39. Flegal KM, Kit BK, Orpana H, Graubard BI. **Association of all-cause mortality with overweight and obesity using standard body mass index categories: a systematic review and meta-analysis.**

JAMA. 2013 Jan 2, 309(1):71-82.

40. Fries WC. **The Natural Diet: Best Foods for Weight Loss, You can eat more and still lose weight.** *WebMD.com* 2013 http://www.webmd.com/diet/features/the-natural-diet-best-foods-for-weight-loss

41. National Center for Chronic Disease Prevention and Health Promotion Division of Nutrition and Physical Activity Research to Practice Series, No. 2 May 2006. **Portion Size: Then and Now.** (CDC website Dec. 2013.) http://www.cdc.gov/nccdphp/dnpa/nutrition/pdf/portion_size_research.pdf

42. Ferreira AV, Generoso SV, Teixeira AL. **Do low-calorie drinks 'cheat' the enteral-brain axis?** *Curr. Opin. Clin. Nutr. Metab. Care.* 2014 Sep. 17(5):465-70.

43. Poulsen SK, Due A, Jordy AB, Kiens B, Stark KD, Stender S, Holst C, Astrup A, Larsen TM. **Health effect of the New Nordic Diet in adults with increased waist circumference: a 6-mo randomized controlled trial.** *Am. J Clin. Nutr.* 2014 Jan. 99(1):35-45.

44. Lera-Orsatti F, Nahas EA, Maestá N, Nahas Neto J, Lera Orsatti C, Vannucchi Portari G, Burini RC. **Effects of resistance training frequency on body composition and metabolics and inflammatory markers in overweight postmenopausal women.** J *Sports Med. Phys. Fitness.* 2014 Jun.; 54(3):317-25.

45. Joseph RP, Casazza K, Durant NH. **The effect of a 3-month moderate-intensity physical activity program on body composition in overweight and obese African American college females.** *Osteoporosis Int.* 2014 Aug 8. [Epub ahead of print]

46. Jakicic JM, Marcus BH, Gallagher KI, Napolitano M, Lang W. **Effect of exercise duration and intensity on weight loss in overweight, sedentary women: a randomized trial.** *JAMA.* 2003 Sep 10; 290(10):1323-30.

47. Rolls BJ. **What is the role of portion control in weight management?** *Int. J Obes. (*Lond). 2014 Jul; 38 Suppl 1:S1-8.

48. Melanson KJ, Summers A, Nguyen V, Brosnahan J, Lowndes J, Angelopoulos TJ, Rippe JM. **Body composition, dietary composition, and components of metabolic syndrome in overweight and obese adults after a 12-week trial on dietary treatments focused on portion control, energy density, or glycemic index.** *Nutr. J.* 2012 Aug 27; 11:57.

49. Webber KH1, Rose SA. **A pilot Internet-based behavioral weight loss intervention with or without commercially available portion-controlled foods.** *Obesity* (Silver Spring). 2013 Sep; 21(9):E354-9.

50. Levitsky DA1, Pacanowski C. **Losing weight without dieting. Use of commercial foods as meal replacements for lunch produces an extended energy deficit.** *Appetite.* 2011 Oct; 57(2):311-7.

51. Hannum SM1, Carson L, Evans EM, Canene KA, Petr EL, Bui L, Erdman JW Jr. **Use of portion-controlled entrees enhances weight loss in women.** *Obes. Res.* 2004 Mar; 12(3):538-46.

52. Willis, FB. *Effective Orthopedic Rehab, Seven Steps to Complete Recovery.* Trafford Publishing, Victoria Canada, 2003

53. Wang L, Lee IM, Manson JE, Buring JE, Sesso HD. **Alcohol consumption, weight gain, and risk of becoming overweight in middle-aged and older women.** *Arch. Intern Med.* 2010 Mar 8; 170(5):453-61.

54. Shin KO, Moritani T. **The combined effects of capsaicin, green tea extract and chicken essence tablets on human autonomic nervous system activity.** *J Nutr. Sci. Vitaminol* (Tokyo). 2007 Apr; 53(2):145-52.

55. Thorsdottir I, Tomasson H, Gunnarsdottir I, Gisladottir E, Kiely M, Parra MD, Bandarra NM, Schaafsma G, Martinéz JA. **Randomized trial of weight-loss-diets for young adults varying in fish and fish oil content.** *Int. J Obes* (Lond). 2007 Oct; 31(10):1560-6.

56. Hill AM, Buckley JD, Murphy KJ, Howe PR. **Combining**

fish-oil supplements with regular aerobic exercise improves body composition and cardiovascular disease risk factors. *Am. J Clin. Nutr.* 2007 May; 85(5):1267-74.

57. Taghizadeh M, Memarzadeh MR, Asemi Z, Esmaillzadeh A. **Effect of the cumin cyminum L. Intake on Weight Loss, Metabolic Profiles and Biomarkers of Oxidative Stress in Overweight Subjects: A Randomized Double-Blind Placebo-Controlled Clinical Trial.** *Ann. Nutr. Metab.* 2015; 66(2-3):117-24.

58. Dulloo AG, Seydoux J, Girardier L, Chantre P, Vandermander J. **Green tea and thermogenesis: interactions between catechin-polyphenols, caffeine and sympathetic activity.** *Int. J Obes. Relat. Metab. Disord.* 2000 Feb; 24(2):252-8.

59. Rosa FT, Freitas EC, Deminice R, Jordão AA, Marchini JS. **Oxidative stress and inflammation in obesity after taurine supplementation: a double-blind, placebo-controlled study.** *Eur. J Nutr.* 2014 Apr; 53(3):823-30.

60. Jeukendrup AE1, Randell R. **Fat burners: nutrition supplements that increase fat metabolism.** *Obes. Rev.* 2011 Oct; 12(10):841-51.

61. Spiegel K, Leproult R, L'Hermite-Balériaux M, Copinschi G, Penev PD, Van Cauter E. **Leptin levels are dependent on sleep duration: relationships with sympathovagal balance, carbohydrate regulation, cortisol, and thyrotropin.** *Journal of Clinical Endocrinology and Metabolism.* 2004; 89(11):5762–5771.

62. Diliberti N, Bordi P, Conklin MT, Roe LS, Rolls BJ. **Increased portion size leads to increased energy intake in a restaurant meal.** *Obes. Res.* 2004; 12: 562–568.

63. Rolls BJ. **What is the role of portion control in weight management?** *International Journal of Obesity* (2014) 38, S1–S8

64. Bezerra IN, Curioni C, Sichieri R. **Association between eating out of home and body weight.** *Nutr. Rev.* 2012; 70: 65–79.

65. Gudzune KA, Doshi RS, Mehta AK, Chaudhry ZW, Jacobs DK, Vakil RM, Lee CJ, Bleich SN, Clark JM. **Efficacy of**

commercial weight-loss programs: an updated system. *Ann. Intern. Med.* 2015 Apr 7; 162(7):501-12.

66. Foster GD, Wadden TA, Lagrotte CA, Vander Veur ᴗ Hesson LA, Homko CJ, et al. A randomized comparison of a commercially available portion-controlled weight-loss intervention with a diabetes self-management education program. *Nutr. Diabetes.* 2013; 3:e63.

67. Figueroa A, Vicil F, Sanchez-Gonzalez MA, Wong A, Ormsbee MJ, Hooshmand S, Daggy B. Effects of diet and/or low-intensity resistance exercise training on arterial stiffness, adiposity, and lean mass in obese postmenopausal women. *Am. J Hypertens.* 2013; 26:416-23.

68. Chen IJ, Liu CY, Chiu JP, Hsu CH. Therapeutic effect of high-dose green tea extract on weight reduction: A randomized, double-blind, placebo-controlled clinical trial. *Clin. Nutr.* 2015 May 29.

69. Azimi P, Ghiasvand R, Feizi A, Hariri M, Abbasi B. Effects of Cinnamon, Cardamom, Saffron, and Ginger Consumption on Markers of Glycemic Control, Lipid Profile, Oxidative Stress, and Inflammation in Type 2 Diabetes Patients. *Rev. Diabet Stud.* 2014 Fall-Winter; 11(3-4):258-66.

70. Mullin GE. Supplements for weight loss: hype or help for obesity? Part II. The inside scoop on green coffee bean extract. *Nutr. Clin. Pract.* 2015 Apr; 30(2):311-2.

71. Osama AJ, Shehab Ael-K. Psychological wellbeing and biochemical modulation in response to weight loss in obese type 2 diabetes patients. *Afr. Health Sci.* 2015 Jun; 15(2):503-12.

72. Mayo Clinic Website (July 2015) http://www.mayoclinic.org/diseases-conditions/arthritis/in-depth/arthritis/ART-20047971

73. John MM, Kalish SR, Perns SV, Willis FB. Dynamic Splinting for Hallux Limitus: a Randomized, Controlled Trial. *J American Podiatric Medical Assoc.* 2011 July/Aug; 101(4):285-88.

Supporting Website Information

(as accessed September 2014 and June 2015)

www.WedMD.com

http://www.Medscape.com/

http://www.cdc.gov/nccdphp/dnpa/nutrition/pdf/
portion_size_research.pdf

http://www.mayoclinic.com/health/water/NU00283

www.HealthyPeople.gov

http://www.cdc.gov/nchs/fastats/overwt.htm

http://health.gov/dietaryguidelines/2010.asp

http://www.LiveStrong.com

www.ChooseMyPlate.gov

http://www.lifescript.com/

American Dietetic Association http://www.eatright.org

US Department of Agriculture Center for Nutrition:
http://www.usda.gov/cnpp

USDA Dietary Guidelines:
http://www.nal.usda.gov/fnic/dga/index.html

The Interactive Food Guide Pyramid:
http://www.nal.usda.gov:8001/py/pmap.htm

Nutrition and Athletic Performance: http://www.ms-se.com

Supplement Information:
http://www.acsm.org/health+fitness/comments.htm

NOTE: A Daily Food Tracking Chart and recipes are online at www.DocWillis.org

BODY SUMMATION SCORE

(See Chapter 2 for instructions on filling this out.)

Today's date _____

Age _____

Physician's name _____ *and*
   approval (Date:_____)

_____ Body weight (Morning weight before eating)
_____ Height in inches
_____ BMI: (Weight pounds ÷ Inches of height) x 10

Girth Measurements:
_____ Neck
_____ Shoulders
_____ Upper Arm
_____ Wrist
_____ Chest
_____ Waist
_____ Hips
_____ Upper thigh (widest girth)
_____ Lower thigh (2" above knee)
_____ Calf
_____ Ankle
_____ Current Dress Size or Coat Size

_____ TOTAL of all amounts

To figure out percentage of change, subtract the total of this score from the previous score. Take that number and divide by previous score. Then multiply the answer by 100.

_____ Percentage of change

ABOUT THE AUTHOR

DOC WILLIS is a weight loss provider and a clinical scientist. After his unsurvivable plane crash, he earned both a Master's degree and PhD in kinesiology before completing his Medical Degree (MBBS) in the British Commonwealth and is a board certified holistic physician. After designing and directing dozens of clinical trials (50 medical publications, 30 scientific presentations, 4 books, and lectures at medical universities from Hawaii to the Netherlands), he was chosen to be a Fellow of the American College of Sports Medicine.

The plane crash that started Doc's second chance resulted in a three year series of 16 sequential operations to rebuild his legs. God gave him victory when he squatted 550 lbs. a few years later! (Matt 19:26) The crash also resulted in a moderately severe brain injury where he lost all manners, math skills, and episodic memories. His rehab resulted in earning four degrees and growing from being a disabled student to beicomng a professor of kinesiology! (Psalm 37:4)

Twelve years ago Doc found himself to be obese at age 40 (due to hypothyroid secretion), which prompted him to explore research on weight loss. He designed the holistic, RightSize™ program, and quickly lost 45 lbs. He has maintained his weight loss for over a decade. Now Doc is preparing to compete in a Senior, Master's Body-builder when he turns 55 in a few years!

You are invited to contact Doc Willis and his team at www.DocWillis.org